Improving Maternal and Child Health Care

A Blueprint for Community Action in the Pittsburgh Region

Harold Alan Pincus, Stephen B. Thomas, Donna J. Keyser, Nicholas Castle,
Jacob W. Dembosky, Ray Firth, Michael D. Greenberg, Nancy Pollock,
Evelyn Reis, Veronica Sansing, Sarah Scholle

Supported by The Heinz Endowments

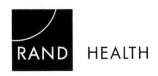

RAND HEALTH

The research described in this report was sponsored by The Heinz Endowments.

Library of Congress Cataloging-in-Publication Data

Improving maternal and child health care : a blueprint for community action in the Pittsburgh region /
Harold Pincus ... [et al.].
    p. cm.
    "MG-225."
    Includes bibliographical references.
    ISBN 0-8330-3717-X (pbk. : alk. paper)
    1. Maternal health services—Pennsylvania—Pittsburgh. 2. Child health services—Pennsylvania—Pittsburgh.
3. Community health services—Pennsylvania—Pittsburgh. 4. Maternal health services—Pennsylvania—Allegheny
County. 5. Child health services—Pennsylvania—Allegheny County. 6. Community health services—
Pennsylvania—Allegheny County.
    [DNLM: 1. Maternal-Child Health Centers—organization & administration—Pennsylvania. 2. Community
Health Services—organization & administration—Pennsylvania. WA 310 1345 2004] I. Pincus, Harold Alan,
1951–

RG961.P4I48 2004
362.198'2'0974885—dc22

                                                                                            2004026544

The RAND Corporation is a nonprofit research organization providing objective analysis and effective solutions that address the challenges facing the public and private sectors around the world. RAND's publications do not necessarily reflect the opinions of its research clients and sponsors.

RAND® is a registered trademark.

Published 2005 by the RAND Corporation
1776 Main Street, P.O. Box 2138, Santa Monica, CA 90407-2138
1200 South Hayes Street, Arlington, VA 22202-5050
201 North Craig Street, Suite 202, Pittsburgh, PA 15213-1516
RAND URL: http://www.rand.org/
To order RAND documents or to obtain additional information, contact
Distribution Services: Telephone: (310) 451-7002;
Fax: (310) 451-6915; Email: order@rand.org

Preface

This report was commissioned by The Heinz Endowments and developed under the auspices of the RAND–University of Pittsburgh Health Institute in partnership with Allegheny County's Department of Health and Department of Human Services. It is intended for a wide range of stakeholders interested in learning how to improve maternal and child health care service delivery and outcomes in their communities. The recommendations are focused on improving health care for mothers and young children from birth to five years of age in the Pittsburgh region, also known as the geographic entity of Allegheny County, Pennsylvania. However, the overall approach could be extended to other populations and counties in southwestern Pennsylvania and beyond. The processes and findings should prove useful to state and local policymakers; health care providers, payers, agencies, and programs; and concerned community stakeholders, including families and other consumers.

The recommendations are based on a series of activities conducted between January 2002 and December 2003, including an extensive website search and a literature review of best practices in maternal and child health care; an analysis of local and state policies impacting maternal and child health care delivery; and interviews with representatives of model national programs, local providers, and mothers and families in the Pittsburgh region. The recommendations were further enhanced and refined through discussions with a local learning collaborative composed of key maternal and child health care stakeholders in the community, as well as several national experts in the field.

Questions and comments about this report are welcome and should be addressed to the principal investigators:

Harold Alan Pincus, MD
Senior Scientist and Director
RAND–University of Pittsburgh Health Institute

Stephen B. Thomas, PhD
Director, Center for Minority Health
University of Pittsburgh

Contents

Tables

Summary

The Challenge

The health and well-being of mothers, infants, and young children are of critical importance, both as reflections of the current health status of individuals, local communities, and the nation as a whole and as predictors of the health of the next generation. Community leaders in the Pittsburgh region, also known as the geographic entity of Allegheny County, Pennsylvania, have long recognized the importance of the family as society's primary institution for supporting healthy child development and have engaged in intensive efforts to develop effective community-based early childhood interventions and support services primarily focused on families. Despite these efforts, there is ample evidence to suggest that widespread improvement of the local maternal and child health care system continues to be of real and immediate importance. In several key areas of health care, mothers and young children in this community are not receiving the health care services they need, and the result is premature illness and preventable death. In the final analysis, the system of service delivery in the Pittsburgh region is less than ideal in many respects, and it can be improved.

In January 2002, The Heinz Endowments commissioned the RAND Corporation and the University of Pittsburgh, in partnership with Allegheny County's Department of Health and Department of Human Services, to establish a learning collaborative of local stakeholders to (1) catalyze new thinking around the best evidence and practice for maternal and child health care; (2) assess the strengths, weaknesses, and barriers to improvement in the current system of maternal and child health care; (3) identify targets for local policy reform; and (4) develop a blueprint for action that would lead to widespread, sustainable systemwide improvements in local maternal and child health care processes and outcomes. The overall approach was informed, in part, by the Healthy People in Healthy Communities movement, which grew out of the Healthy People 2000 national health-promotion and disease-prevention campaign. This movement seeks to advance the health of communities by forming local coalitions, creating a vision, and measuring results (U.S. Department of Health and Human Services website, http:// www.hhs.gov).

This report provides an overview of the community-based approach through which this work was undertaken, highlights key study findings, and outlines a vision, strategy, and action plan for improving maternal and child health care in the community. This work, which was completed in December 2003, does not represent a predetermined end-state or product; rather, it is an ongoing process of community collaboration and learning.

Mobilizing a Community Collaborative for Change

At the outset of this initiative, the project team recognized that a successful systems-improvement strategy would require a coalition of key individuals and organizations working together to achieve common goals. Therefore, at the initiative's inception, a local stakeholders' learning collaborative was established that brought together people who control the system with people who had lost all hope in the system.

Members of the collaborative represent all key maternal and child health care organizations in the community, including Allegheny County's Department of Health and Department of Human Services, the Children's Cabinet of Allegheny County, local managed-care organizations (MCOs), large provider groups, faith-based organizations, community centers, and families (a list of the members is presented in Appendix A). The full learning collaborative met on a quarterly basis from January 2002 through October 2003, working with the project team in both an advisory and a participatory capacity, and individual members were integrally involved in many of the research tasks of the project.

Given the breadth of the issues involved in health care systems improvement, the first task of the initiative was to identify the areas of greatest need for pregnant women and for children from birth to five years of age in the community. The four priority areas and two best-practice domains identified are shown in Table S.1.

This prioritization of areas and best-practice domains in maternal and child health care provided a useful focus for subsequent data collection, analyses, and discussions regarding policy and practice improvement.

Table S.1
Priority Areas and Best-Practice Domains

Priority Areas for Improvement	Best-Practice Domains
• Prenatal care	• Family engagement
• Family behavioral health	• Care coordination/service integration
• Nutrition	
• Chronic illness and special-care needs	

Barriers and Issues Faced by Families in the Community

To gain a better understanding of the strengths and weaknesses of the local maternal and child health care system, the project team and the learning collaborative considered it essential to listen to the consumers who are attempting to access needed services for their children and families while at the same time dealing with other fundamental life challenges, such as obtaining stable housing, food, and transportation. Consumer members of the learning collaborative identified a subset of families representing different racial and ethnic groups and communities in the Pittsburgh region who could describe both positive and negative experiences with aspects of the local health care system related to the four priority areas.

In a few cases, parents found local agency and program staff to be supportive and helpful, and families were able to develop positive relationships with their care providers. At the same time, several common themes emerged across the families that elucidate important limitations of the current system. These include:

- Difficulty accessing available services
- Racial and economic discrimination in the health care system
- The challenge of dealing with health care problems in the context of other basic needs
- Competition among agencies providing services for children

The families interviewed demonstrated courage in sharing their stories. They told of painful experiences and described efforts to be resourceful and independent in spite of tremendous needs. Despair and hopelessness are common responses when faced with the "Everest-like mountain" that health care delivery systems have become. What can be done to help families scale this mountain? Families recommended the following directions for change:

- Improve access
- Enhance coordination
- Adopt a family-centered approach to service delivery
- Instill and assure respect for families

Barriers and Issues Faced by Local Providers and Program Staff

Ongoing discussions between the project team and the learning collaborative revealed that many local maternal and child health care programs and providers face numerous barriers in their attempts to improve outcomes for mothers with young children. Following the recommendations of learning collaborative members and other community leaders, the project team interviewed 16 local maternal and child health care providers and payers, including county MCOs (listed in Appendix B), to further elucidate these barriers and to uncover possible strategies for overcoming them.

Through this process, the project team identified several barriers to engaging families at the local program level, including:

- Lack of skills, numbers, and types of staff (e.g., nurses)
- Funding limitations and licensing geared to individual patient service
- Factors impacting provider/family relationships
- Lack of transportation to services and programs

The project team also identified a number of issues in coordinating care and integrating services, including:

- Lack of skills, numbers, and types of staff (e.g., care coordinators, behavioral health specialists)
- Organizational "silos" (i.e., vertical organizational structures) created by funding and licensing regulations

- Weak relationships among providers
- Lack of information
- Poor linkages across programs and services

To overcome these barriers, providers and program staff recommended the following directions for change:

- Strengthen provider and staff skills
- Enhance linkages and support relationships among agencies and providers
- Improve access to information
- Consider new types of reimbursement strategies

Lessons Learned from Promising National and Local Programs

From a review of the published literature and information on the Internet, the project team identified 12 promising national and local maternal and child health care programs that provide family-centered care and pursue program coordination or integration in a variety of ways (the programs are listed in Appendix C). Members of the project team interviewed representatives of these programs to determine common strategies or practices that might be useful and relevant to local systems-improvement efforts for engaging families and coordinating care or integrating services. These common strategies and practices are summarized in Table S.2.

The project team's interviews also suggested that funding family-engagement activities and care-coordination/service-integration efforts is difficult and requires some creativity. Several programs braid funds from disparate streams to pay for these activities. Others rely primarily on demonstration grants to cover the expenses. Common funding sources include IDEA Part C; Early and Periodic Screening, Diagnosis and Treatment (EPSDT); Title V, Maternal and Child Health Block Grants; tobacco-settlement funds; state general-revenue funds; Temporary Assistance for Needy Families (TANF); demonstration grants.

Table S.2
Common Strategies and Practices for Engaging Families and Coordinating Care/Integrating Services

Strategies and Practices for Family Engagement	Strategies and Practices for Care Coordination/ Service Integration
• Treatment models that focus on families' strengths	• Use of multidisciplinary treatment teams
• Strong relationships with families and across programs	• Cross-training of staff
• Home-visiting programs	• Integrated information resources
• Locating staff in places that low-income families frequent	• Personal relationships between program directors and program staff
• Involvement of parents in the development of their service plans	• Strong leadership from agency directors

Potential Policy Levers for Enhancing Local Improvement Efforts

Any effort to improve maternal and child health care systems must take into account the full network of government programs and regulations that impact these systems. While there are numerous opportunities for maternal and child health care policy reform at the federal level, the project team focused on identifying the state-level policy changes that would be most likely to enhance local improvement efforts. These policy levers include the following:

- Addressing the negative impact of privacy regulations on the maternal and child health care system by revising the rules to facilitate treatment communication between mental health/substance-abuse treatment providers and other providers, as well as between providers for different family members
- Setting standards that guarantee public transportation for families seeking access to maternal and child health care through Medical Assistance Transportation Program (MATP) services
- Bridging the schism between physical and mental health formalized by the state's Medicaid waiver by requiring that state laws and state Medicaid contracts mandate communication and information-sharing regarding maternal and child health care services across physical and behavioral health care systems and between physical and behavioral health MCOs
- Building mechanisms for collaboration among state and local departments that share responsibility for children, mothers, and families in order to simplify procedures regarding families' access to benefits and services and to reduce the burden of legal/administrative requirements and regulations on providers

While much of the regulatory control for maternal and child health care in the Pittsburgh region rests in the Pennsylvania state capitol of Harrisburg, significant resources are managed locally by leaders who are motivated to improve outcomes for families with young children and who are knowledgeable about providers in the county. Allegheny County's Department of Health and Department of Human Services, as well as the local Medicaid MCOs, play an important role and should be recognized as additional leverage points for improving maternal and child health care programs and services in the region.

A Blueprint for Community Action

Clearly, any effort to confront the multiple issues impacting the overall maternal and child health care system will require a vision of tremendous breadth and power that originates from the community's own needs, values, and goals. This vision, in turn, must inform an ongoing change strategy that reflects the broad array of critical factors and influences that determine the health of individuals, families, and communities. To be achievable and sustainable over the long term, the strategy must drive an action plan that encompasses significant and widespread changes in consciousness and practice; unprecedented cooperation among federal, state, and local governments and between and among the different departments and agencies within these organizations; new types of public-private partnerships to leverage existing infrastructure supports; resources to reduce disparities in access and quality of care; and public education and engagement campaigns that attempt to change public attitudes and standards, educate community residents, and support community-based interventions.

Vision

Members of the Pittsburgh region's learning collaborative have identified the following key components of their shared vision for achieving an outstanding local maternal and child health care system:

- Promote healthy lifestyles and positive health outcomes
- Reduce preventable disease and environmental health risks
- Eliminate health disparities
- Ensure access to quality care for young children, mothers, and families

Ideally, such a system will have the following characteristics:

- An established medical or social service home[1] or homes for each family in the community and/or each mother and her child(ren)
- A family-centered, culturally competent approach to care, in which providers address the needs of and draw on the strengths of the entire family being served
- Integrated/holistic services, with service providers working closely together, addressing all aspects of a family's health and social needs that affect the at-risk child
- A high-quality maternal and child health care workforce, well trained in the principles of family-centeredness, cultural competence, and integrated/holistic care
- Families well educated about available programs and resources and about healthy behaviors (e.g., proper nutrition, the importance of prenatal care, smoking cessation, reducing environmental health risks) and empowered to demand high-quality maternal and child health care
- Effective leadership at the state and county levels, with clear lines of authority and accountability for performance

Strategy

To achieve this vision, a RAND–University of Pittsburgh project team, in collaboration with local leaders of the maternal and child health care system, will:

- Expand and further engage the existing local maternal and child health care stakeholders' learning collaborative to form a *leadership collaborative* with the power and authority to establish priorities; mobilize available resources; guide and support community-based quality-improvement interventions; measure outcomes; and advocate for change in policy, financing, and practice at the state and local levels
- Advance a *family-centered approach* to maternal and child health care that (1) establishes a medical or social service home or homes for each family in the community

---

[1] A medical or social service home provides the patient and her family with a broad spectrum of care over a period of time and coordinates all of the care they receive.

and/or each mother and her child(ren); (2) recognizes a family's strengths, while seeking to understand and meet its basic and other health care needs; and (3) is nurtured in an environment of cultural competency and trusting, respectful relationships

- Promote effective *coordination and integration of care and outreach*, particularly between and among physical health care, behavioral health care, environmental health programs, and social support services
- Develop plans to establish *countywide integrated data systems* that (1) provide useful information on available services and resources for families, (2) support practitioners' efforts to coordinate care and track a family's progress across agencies and programs, (3) enable agencies to monitor service utilization and performance across individual programs, and (4) support health plans in developing flexible, performance-based payment structures that ensure provision of needed services and drive quality-improvement efforts at the provider and practitioner levels

Action Plan

Outlined below is an action plan for the Pittsburgh region that should be implemented by specific stakeholder groups at various levels of the maternal and child health care system, with the local stakeholders' leadership collaborative serving as the organizing entity:

- At the *state/local policy level*, the action plan will expand engagement of community stakeholders; improve the dissemination of information on maternal and child health care programs, services, and resources; build the community's capacity to monitor health outcomes for provider accountability and quality improvement; target specific areas for regulatory, licensing, and other policy reform; and enhance advocacy for improving maternal and child health care.
- At the *payer/plan level*, the action plan will promote the design of financial and other incentives that ensure provision of needed services and drive quality-improvement efforts at the provider and practitioner levels.
- At the *agency/program/provider* level, the action plan will establish new types of training, strategies, and practice that result in increased family engagement and care coordination.

Toward a Model Maternal and Child Health Care System in the Pittsburgh Region

To bring this blueprint for action to life, between January 2004 and December 2005, the project team will conduct a policy- and practice-improvement demonstration in the Pittsburgh region that will operate under the direction of an expanded stakeholders' leadership collaborative. The goal of the demonstration will be to begin building a model maternal and child health care system that will lead to improved health care for mothers and young children in the region.

At the *policy level*, the project team will:

- Organize two policy working groups to develop plans for (1) integrated countywide data collection, analysis, and dissemination of information on maternal and child health care service utilization and outcomes; and (2) flexible, performance-based payment mechanisms that reward quality improvement
- Support the leadership collaborative in its efforts to tailor and implement proposed policy changes in the Pittsburgh region

At the *practice level*, the project team will:

- Create and support at least two community-based practice-improvement teams that will (1) involve strategic partnerships among local payers/plans, programs, and families in previously designated high-risk communities; (2) gather baseline information on specific indicators related to the key priority areas of prenatal care, nutrition, behavioral health, chronic illness, and special-care needs, with linkages to environmental health; (3) adopt and test proven processes and practices for increasing family engagement and care coordination in accordance with the plan-act-study-do rapid-cycle quality-improvement model; and (4) develop data systems and financing mechanisms to support these practice improvements
- Monitor and evaluate the progress of the community-based practice-improvement teams, basing the evaluation on process and outcomes data provided by the individual teams, as well as changes on key indicators of family engagement and care coordination measured first at baseline and then at the completion of the action plans
- Synthesize the information from the evaluation into a community report card documenting the progress of the community-based practice-improvement teams
- Develop a countywide plan for the sustainability and diffusion of quality-improvement strategies that are shown to enhance maternal and child health care

The primary outcomes of this policy and practice improvement demonstration will be:

- A local leadership collaborative structure and process for improving policy and practice components of the maternal and child health care system that have been identified as priorities by community stakeholders
- Communitywide plans for (1) integrated data collection, analysis, and dissemination of information on maternal and child health care service utilization and outcomes; and (2) flexible, performance-based payment mechanisms; both of these plans will incorporate strategies for overcoming anticipated barriers
- Community-based practice-improvement teams that have demonstrated and documented their success
- Mechanisms that will enable the sustainability and diffusion of the improvement process

Generalizability to Other Communities

Recognizing that communities differ markedly with respect to their history, demographics, economy, and governance, it is uncertain whether the community-based collaborative process undertaken in the Pittsburgh region could take hold as effectively in other areas. Certainly, to a large degree, the success of this process locally will be attributable to the historical importance of the family in the community, the energy and cohesiveness of community leadership, and the ability to mobilize significant resources to support visionary change.

At the same time, the idea of creating healthy communities is gaining momentum across cities and counties both nationwide and around the world. Although, in most cases, these communities have identified goals and pursued action plans related to issues other than maternal and child health care, they share many of the same characteristics with the Pittsburgh region, including a common vision, a willingness to work collaboratively, a free flow of information among all major stakeholders in the community, and clear opportunities for improvement. In this sense, Pittsburgh's specific experience in designing a community blueprint for action should prove useful to a range of communities, regardless of the goals they are pursuing.

For those seeking improvement in maternal and child health care in particular, or in service delivery to families in poverty more generally, many of the best practices, barriers, and potential solutions presented in this report could serve as a basis for developing a community-based collaborative approach designed specifically to address their communities' needs.

Acknowledgments

This report would not have been possible without the guidance, input, and vision of the Pittsburgh region's maternal and child health care learning collaborative. The willingness of collaborative members to participate in this study reflects their ongoing commitment to seeking creative approaches for improving maternal and child health care outcomes in the community. The RAND–University of Pittsburgh project team looks forward to the collaborative's continuing involvement in efforts to implement the community action plan outlined herein.

Many others outside of the learning collaborative also made important contributions to this study. The authors acknowledge with appreciation the representatives of the national and local maternal and child health care agencies and programs who participated in telephone interviews and site visits. We also express our deep gratitude to the mothers and family members in the community who invited members of the project team and the learning collaborative into their homes to complete the in-depth family interviews. Their input has enabled this report to give voice to the concerns and hopes of local parents and other caregivers who have demonstrated courage and resilience in the face of real and perceived barriers to providing their children with a nurturing environment for healthy growth and development.

This work was made possible through the financial support of The Heinz Endowments and the ongoing commitment of Program Director Margaret Petruska and Program Officer Carmen Anderson for Children, Youth and Families. Their interest in improving the health and well-being of young children in the Pittsburgh region has motivated the community to develop and implement a new vision for delivering quality health care to all families, especially those most in need.

CHAPTER ONE

Introduction

The Challenge

The health and well-being of mothers, infants, and young children are of critical importance, both as reflections of the current health status of individuals, local communities, and the nation as a whole and as predictors of the health of the next generation. As recent child-development research has shown, the opportunities and challenges for promoting a child's long-term physical health and social and emotional growth are most significant in the early years, from birth to five years of age, when access to high-quality maternal and child health care services takes on special importance, especially for people who live with the burdens of poverty, racism, and social isolation. At the same time, as evidenced by the continued nationwide disparities in health care outcomes, efforts to reach these populations have had, at best, mixed results, in the Pittsburgh region as well as elsewhere.

About the Pittsburgh Region

The Pittsburgh region, also known as the geographic entity of Allegheny County, is located in southwestern Pennsylvania, and Pittsburgh is the county seat. According to 2000 U.S. Census data, 1,281,666 people, 537,150 households, and 332,495 families reside in the county. Twenty-six percent of the households include children under the age of 18; 46 percent are married couples living together; 12 percent have a woman whose husband does not live with her; and 38 percent are non-families. The racial makeup of the county is 84 percent white, 12 percent African-American, and 4 percent other races. The median age is 40 years, with 22 percent of the population under the age of 18. Median household income is $37,267 (U.S. median income is $37,005); 11 percent of the residents live below the poverty level (compared with 13 percent for the nation as a whole); and 17 percent of the children live below the poverty level (compared with 20 percent for the nation as a whole).

The Pittsburgh region is rich in health care resources. There are many excellent hospitals and an academic medical center, numerous health clinics and programs in low-income communities, and local foundations that actively support efforts to enhance health care delivery and outcomes. The Allegheny County Health Department manages Title V Maternal and Child Health and related programs, such as the Women, Infants and Children's (WIC's) Supplemental Nutrition Program and the Childhood Lead Poisoning Prevention Program. The Pennsylvania Department of Health (DOH) is responsible for many of these programs at the state level. Counties in Pennsylvania manage many of the federal and state-funded social services for the Pennsylvania Department of Public Welfare (DPW), including programs such as child welfare, early intervention (Part C), and mental health and substance-abuse treatment services. To deliver these services, the Pittsburgh region has made significant use of nonprofit agencies and has a relatively large network of private service providers. The Pennsylvania DPW has contracted with three physical health managed-care organizations (MCOs) to serve Allegheny County citizens on Medicaid, while Medicaid-funded mental health and substance-abuse treatment services are "carved out." The state contracts with the county to manage these services and to facilitate coordination with other services, such as child welfare and early intervention. Allegheny County contracts with a local behavioral health MCO to manage contracting with service providers and to assure access.

Building on a Legacy of Community Leadership and Engagement

Community leaders in the Pittsburgh region have long recognized the importance of the family as society's primary institution for supporting healthy child development and have engaged in intensive efforts to develop effective community-based early-childhood interventions and support services. Here and throughout this report, the term "family" refers to any combination of primary caregiver and child living in the same household, although the primary focus is on mothers and children from birth to five years of age.

The Pittsburgh region has been well served by community mobilization of resources and organizational commitments to resolve a number of challenges, especially those faced by families living in poverty. For example, the Healthy Start Program, which started as a communitywide demonstration in 1991, can be credited with lowering the infant mortality rate by 47 percent in its project areas (54 Pittsburgh neighborhoods and four other county municipalities). There has been a 4 percent decrease in babies with low birth weight and a 21 percent decrease in babies with very low birth weight. Births where the mother received late or no prenatal care have been reduced by 46 percent since the baseline period (Allegheny County Health Department, On-line Health Beat). The Healthy Start Program provides credible evidence that health care leaders in the Pittsburgh region know what works and how to deploy effective programs in areas of greatest need.

More recently, the Allegheny County Health Department Maternal and Child Health Bureau and Healthy Start have initiated a continuous quality-improvement process to analyze fetal/infant mortality and to mobilize the community to address this problem in a targeted fashion (Allegheny County Health Department, On-line Health Reports). Additionally, the Birth to Five Committee of the Children's Cabinet, organized under the auspices of the Allegheny County Human Services Department in the fall of 2002, has recommended a number of strategies for serving families with young children, strategies that utilize child care, family support, mental health, child welfare, early intervention, and drug- and alcohol-abuse public services (Children's Cabinet, 2002).

Ongoing Need for Systemwide Improvement

Despite these efforts, there is ample evidence to suggest that widespread improvement of the local maternal and child health care system continues to be of real and immediate importance. In several key areas of health care, mothers and young children in the community are not receiving the health care services they need, and the result is premature illness and death.

The Allegheny County Department of Health collects data on eight maternal and child health care indicators established as Healthy People 2010 (HP 2010) objectives by the U.S. Department of Health and Human Services. The good news is that Allegheny County meets two important HP 2010 objectives, as shown in Table 1.1. However, more work is needed because the county fails to meet six other HP 2010 objectives, as shown in Table 1.2.

The result of the county's failure to meet these objectives means that of the 14,249 infants born in Allegheny County in 2000, 1,159 (8.1 percent) were born at low birth weight; 257 (1.8 percent) were born at very low birth weight; and more than 100 infants died (Allegheny County Health Department, 1999, 2000a,b). Additionally, the data clearly expose the gap between black and white babies, with African-Americans bearing a disproportionate burden. For example, while the county met the HP 2010 objective of at least 90 percent of *all mothers* receiving early prenatal care in 2000, 1,151 mothers (8.3 percent of known cases) went without early prenatal care, 39 percent of whom were black. In other words, 17.3 percent of all black mothers did not receive early prenatal care.

The scientific literature on child development is conclusive regarding the negative lifelong consequences of low birth weight and lack of prenatal care. These babies are at increased risk for significant delays in their social and emotional development and are likely to experience other challenging behaviors as they grow. Research shows that 10 to 25 percent of the low-birth-weight infants will show evidence of detrimental development (Powell, Fixsen, and Dunlap, 2003).

The data also suggest that solutions to maternal and child health care must address the broader social issues that sustain these disparities in health. For example, according to an annual study by The Annie E. Casey Foundation, of the 50 largest cities in the United States, Pittsburgh has the highest reported rate of maternal smoking (23.3 percent) (Annie E.

Table 1.1
Healthy People 2010 Objectives Met by Allegheny County

Indicator	Allegheny County	HP 2010 Objective
Total infant mortality rate per 1,000 live births	7	7
Early prenatal care for all mothers as a percentage of live births	91.7	90

Table 1.2
Healthy People 2010 Objectives Not Met by Allegheny County

Indicator	Allegheny County	HP 2010 Objective
Black infant mortality rate per 1,000 live births	16.6	11
Low birth weight for black infants as a percentage of live births	14	9
Low birth weight for all infants as a percentage of live births	7.5	5
Very low birth weight for black infants as a percentage of live births	3.9	0.9
Very low birth weight for all infants as a percentage of live births	1.8	0.9
Early prenatal care for all mothers as a percentage of live births	82.7	90

Casey Foundation, 1999); in comparison, the average reported national rate is 9.6 percent. In Allegheny County, 17 percent of women who gave birth reported smoking during pregnancy. Pittsburgh and Allegheny County have held this high ranking for nine of the last 10 years (Tobacco Free Allegheny). The Allegheny County Department of Human Services estimates that 75 percent of families involved in Children and Youth Services have some disease of addiction. Moreover, many minority children living in low-income inner-city homes experience disproportionately higher morbidity and mortality due to chronic illnesses, such as asthma. These children may be more sensitive than others to harmful environmental factors, including atmospheric pollution and second-hand smoke (Sunyer et al., 1993; Gortmaker et al., 1982).

There is also evidence that mothers and young children in Allegheny County suffer from lack of food and inadequate nutrition. The Greater Pittsburgh Community Food Bank provides food assistance to an average of 59,477 people each week. Approximately 46 percent of those served are black, and 7.2 percent of the members of households served are children under five years of age. More than three-quarters (76.7 percent) of the households with children served by the Food Bank lack secure access to nutritious food, and 38.7 percent routinely experience hunger (Myoung, Ohls, and Cohen, 2001).

Clearly, the poor health outcomes of mothers and children cannot be addressed in isolation from the broader social context in which babies are born and families live. A systems approach to improving maternal and child health care would result not only in obvious health benefits for families and children but also in significant cost savings for federal and state governments and other purchasers of health care who are currently struggling with tight budgets and substantial deficits. The costs associated with poor maternal and child health outcomes are substantial. In one recent study, for example, the average cost of caring for a very low-birth-weight infant in the first year of life was estimated at $59,730, while the cost of proper prenatal care and nutrition that can prevent infants from being born severely underweight is relatively inexpensive (Rogowski, 1998). Some researchers have found that 10 percent of all health care costs for children are attributable to low birth weight (e.g., Lewitt et al., 1995). Nicholson et al. (2000) estimated that the nationwide incremental costs of additional tests, procedures, and physician fees in the management of preterm labor and care for premature infants after birth amounted to $459 million each year. It has also been estimated that passive second-hand smoke exposure among children results in direct annual medical expenditures in the United States of $4.6 billion (Aligne and Stoddard, 1997).

Designing an Innovative Approach to Improving Maternal and Child Health Care

The Pittsburgh region has made and is continuing to make progress in improving the local system of maternal and child health care. The county has model programs of exceptional quality and professional staff and administrators who are dedicated to serving all members of the community. However, the continued evidence of poor health outcomes and racial disparities cannot be discounted. In the final analysis, the local system of service delivery is less than ideal in many respects, and it can be improved.

In January 2002, The Heinz Endowments commissioned the RAND Corporation and the University of Pittsburgh, in partnership with Allegheny County's Department of

Health and Department of Human Services, to establish a learning collaborative of local stakeholders to (1) catalyze new thinking around the best evidence and practice for maternal and child health care; (2) assess the strengths, weaknesses, and barriers to improvement in the current system of maternal and child health care; (3) identify targets for local policy reform; and (4) develop a blueprint for action that would lead to widespread, sustainable systemwide improvements in local maternal and child health care processes and outcomes. The overall approach was informed, in part, by the Healthy People in Healthy Communities movement, which grew out of the Healthy People 2000 national health-promotion and disease-prevention campaign. This movement seeks to advance the health of communities by forming local coalitions, creating a vision, and measuring results (U.S. Department of Health and Human Services, n.d.). The stakeholders' learning collaborative that was established in the Pittsburgh region brought together people who control the system with people who had lost all hope in the system, resulting in many innovative ideas worthy of exploration.

This report provides an overview of the community-based approach through which this work was undertaken; highlights key findings from local family stakeholders and providers; identifies best practices that have been successful in model national programs; suggests potential policy levers for enhancing local improvement efforts; and outlines a vision, strategy, and action plan for improving maternal and child health care in the Pittsburgh region. This work, which was completed in December 2003, does not represent a predetermined end-state or product; rather, it is an ongoing process of community collaboration and learning.

Mobilizing a Community Collaborative for Change

At the outset of this initiative, the project team recognized that a successful systems-improvement strategy would require a coalition of key individuals and organizations working together to achieve common goals. Community partnerships, particularly those that involve nontraditional partners, can be among the most effective tools for improving the health of communities (Healthy People 2010, n.d.). Community leaders who demonstrate energy, commitment, and willingness to collaborate with others can inspire and sustain action. Local community organizations, by virtue of their influence, resources, and involvement in the community and the respect they command, can support needed actions and mobilize resources to help implement those actions. Equally important is the involvement of consumers and parents who engage directly with the health care system to provide their children and families with the care they need.

Establishment and Operation of the Learning Collaborative

The local stakeholders' learning collaborative was established at the initiative's inception. Members of the collaborative represent all key maternal and child health care organizations in the community, including Allegheny County's Department of Health and Department of Human Services, the Children's Cabinet of Allegheny County, local MCOs, large provider groups, faith-based organizations, community centers, and families. Engagement of families was an integral part of the learning process. Three family representatives from the community served on the collaborative, providing input to the development of the interview protocol for families, identifying families in the community to interview about their personal experiences with the health care system, and serving as primary family interviewers after receiving formal training in the conduct of qualitative interviews. The members of the learning collaborative and their organizational affiliations are listed in Appendix A.

The full learning collaborative met on a quarterly basis from January 2002 through October 2003, working with the project team in both an advisory and a participatory capacity. Individual members were integrally involved in many of the research tasks of the project, including initial priority setting and task formulation; identifying national and local programs for study; developing interview protocols; and participating in national and local program interviews. Each of the critical steps in the process was guided by the experiences and input of the collaborative members through periodic formal surveys, informal feedback loops, and small-group meetings. Table 2.1 summarizes the tasks and timing of the key steps in this collaborative process.

Table 2.1
Timetable of Key Steps in the Collaborative Process

January 2002	First meeting to review goals of initiative and refine tasks and timeline
April 2002	Second meeting to review identification of priority areas and best-practice domains, issues and concerns of families as related to those areas and domains, and key policy areas of relevance to maternal and child health care
July 2002	Third meeting to refine interview protocols for families and programs, finalize list of interviewees, and review progress of policy analysis
November 2002	Fourth meeting to share lessons from the field on family engagement and care coordination/service integration, with special consideration of issues and concerns raised by family and program representatives
February 2003	Fifth meeting to review preliminary findings from family and program interviews and to discuss state policy leverage points
June 2003	One-day retreat to develop key components of systems-improvement plan for maternal and child health care in Pittsburgh and Allegheny County
October 2003	Sixth meeting to review and finalize community blueprint for action

Setting a Direction for Change

Given the breadth of the issues involved in health care systems improvement, the first task of the initiative was to identify the areas of greatest need for pregnant women and for children from birth to five years of age in the community. After the first meeting of the collaborative, the project team developed a survey to help identify the most critical maternal and child health care issues in the Pittsburgh region. The survey, in combination with the Maternal and Child Health Needs Assessment 2001 from the Allegheny County Health Department and the Allegheny County Health Department Analysis of Healthy People 2000/2010 Goals, identified four priority areas for improvement in maternal and child health, as shown in Table 2.2. A number of important issues (e.g., health disparities) were addressed across the four priority areas, while others (e.g., lack of services, lack of insurance) were integrated into one or more areas.

Drawing on the findings of an extensive literature review of the evidence on best practices in maternal and child health care, the project team also identified two key domains of best practice and related features, as shown in Table 2.3. This prioritization of areas and best-practice domains in maternal and child health care provided a useful focus for subsequent data collection, analyses, and discussions regarding policy and practice improvement.

Table 2.2
Priority Areas for Improvement

- Prenatal care
- Family behavioral health
- Nutrition
- Chronic illness and special-care needs

Table 2.3
Domains of Best Practice and Related Features

Family Engagement	Care Coordination/Service Integration
• Focus on the family as the unit of service	• Provision of a holistic array of services, or at least meaningful linkages across programs and services
• An effective outreach component for supporting at-risk mothers and children	
• Culturally competent staff	• Effective mechanisms to help families navigate the health care system
• Programs and services tailored to the needs and strengths of families	

Laying the Groundwork for Change

"We must move from thinking in silo fashion to integrated planning and operations. Without integrated service delivery, too many individuals fall through the cracks while trying to navigate the often confusing and very different systems for meeting their needs."

Pennsylvania Secretary of Public Welfare Estelle Richman

The members of the learning collaborative contributed to and became engaged with the work of the project team as each component of the approach was formulated, designed, carried out, and synthesized. Their ideas and perspectives have served as a useful filter for understanding and making relevant to the Pittsburgh region diverse information culled from extensive research and data-collection activities.

This shared learning process culminated in a one-day retreat held on June 2, 2003, where the collaborative members worked together to develop the key elements of a systems-improvement plan for maternal and child health care. Pennsylvania Secretary of Public Welfare Estelle Richman served as the keynote speaker. The objectives identified at the retreat, along with the strategies for achieving them, formed the basis for the community action plan to overcome key systems barriers. The plan, described in Chapter Seven, builds on existing community resources and infrastructure, reflects best evidence and practice, and addresses both policy issues and family and local program concerns. It is designed to achieve important, sustainable, and replicable improvements in the health care delivery system for mothers and children in the Pittsburgh region.

CHAPTER THREE

Barriers and Issues Faced by Families in the Community

To gain a better understanding of the strengths and weaknesses of the local maternal and child health care system, the project team and the learning collaborative considered it essential to listen to the consumers who are attempting to access needed services for their children and families while at the same time dealing with other fundamental life challenges, such as obtaining stable housing, food, and transportation. Consumer members of the learning collaborative identified a subset of families representing different racial and ethnic groups and communities in the Pittsburgh region who could describe both positive and negative experiences with aspects of the local health care system related to the four priority areas. Since the focus of this initiative is on improving the local system of maternal and child health care, only primary caregivers who are mothers were interviewed. As the initiative moves forward, it will be important to identify the issues and concerns of fathers who serve as primary caregivers and to integrate appropriate strategies for addressing their issues and concerns in the community's overall action plan.

A selection of family stories is presented below. In a few cases, parents found local agency and program staff to be supportive and helpful, and families were able to develop positive relationships with providers. At the same time, several common themes emerged across families that elucidate important limitations of the current system. While the examples provided do not encompass the full range of experiences encountered by the many different local consumers seeking maternal and child health care, they serve as a useful starting point for identifying some of the major problems that need to be addressed if improvements are to

---

A Mother's Story

An African-American grandmother in her sixties who is overweight, diabetic, and has cardiovascular disease lives with her husband and three grandchildren in a lower-middle-class neighborhood. Her poor health makes it difficult to take care of both herself and her grandchildren. *"I tell [the doctors], by the time I'm finished taking care of three kids, I don't have the energy. All I want to do is go to sleep. So they're aware of it. They just forget it. They conveniently forget."* The grandson and granddaughters she cares for do not qualify for free health insurance because their father's income exceeds the maximum-income limitations. She and her husband make little money, and the children could qualify for health care if the grandparents were legal guardians, but the father would not allow this. *"The services that I could be linked with will not take care of me and the children because their father's income is too great."* She needs help keeping the children healthy, but the only way she can get help is by taking them to the emergency room. She has difficulty getting help from agencies because she does not know who to contact and what services will benefit her the most. *"Before HMOs, I never had a problem. After HMOs, I have a whole lot of problems."*

---

be made. The chapter concludes with a summary of the directions for change recommended by families. The project team and the learning collaborative drew on these recommendations when formulating the blueprint for action presented in Chapter Seven.

Accessing the System

> *"I guess it's a matter of knowing where to go and who to contact . . . it's just really frustrating . . . I see a lot of parents with children who do not have health insurance having to jump through hoops to get the services that they need for their children."*
>
> Mother and provider-agency board member, Allegheny County

Families reported significant problems identifying and obtaining services for themselves and their children. Several mothers mentioned looking through the telephone book and calling various agencies to obtain help. No mention was made of existing online services designed to centralize access to providers (e.g., the United Way website). Participants expressed frustration over the inability of agency staff to provide more help and said that the help staff did provide was often confusing or insufficient. One staff person told a mother that she was not eligible for the Women, Infants and Children (WIC) program, while another told that same mother that she *was* eligible. The mother did not know how to apply for the program, and the agency she went to did little to help her. Another mother talked about the difficulties she had finding help to deal with her drug problem. She said that she paged through the telephone book looking for services, and when she found a program and received an evaluation, she was told that her habit was "not serious enough" and was turned away. As a result, her drug habit worsened.

Prejudice, Stereotyping, and Disrespect

> *"I was in a homeless shelter. I believe that had a lot to do with it [the poor quality of care she received]. . . . They judged me for being down there. They judged me for how many kids I had."*
>
> Mother, Allegheny County

Families recounted stark examples of racial and economic discrimination in the health care system. One white woman attributed the callous and neglectful treatment she received during pregnancy to negative stereotypes and judgments made by providers because the father of her baby was an African-American. This same mother believed that health care professionals did not provide thorough care for her when a possible miscarriage was identified. Families also felt they received poor treatment because they relied on public assistance programs. Several families described feeling that health care professionals did not show respect for them as parents and for their knowledge of their children's needs. One mother felt that service providers undermined her role as a parent.

A Mother's Story

A single African-American mother in her late thirties or early forties lives with her very young foster daughter in a lower-middle-income neighborhood in close proximity to an industrial coke factory, which exacerbates the child's asthma. This mother believes that health care professionals have treated her poorly because she is on Medicaid. *"The doctor that I was dealing with, he just had the worst bed-side manner . . . no one [should] talk down to me, you know . . . because I have welfare insurance. And that's the way I felt. It was like we were second-rate citizens."* But she has also made valuable contacts with agency staff who have helped her figure out who to contact and where to go for help. She found a doctor who was genuinely concerned about her daughter's health and enrolled her in a research study that provided medication. *"[My daughter] just thinks he is the coolest doctor in the world. And he thinks she is just the coolest kid in the world. But that was the one good experience I had."* She also found a program for her daughter that sent regular reminders for checkups, which was a great help to her. The mother is now a very active member on a local provider agency's board, helping others who are experiencing the same problems she experienced.

Families Face Competing Demands

"Sometimes professionals don't understand that even though you wanted to make a doctor's appointment, you needed to go get food."

Mother, Allegheny County

Several families described the challenges of dealing with health care problems in the context of other basic needs, such as obtaining stable housing, food, and transportation. They reported that health care staff often showed little understanding of how "the little things" made seemingly simple steps in getting and following through with care quite difficult. Providers often fail to recognize the competing demands that families face. Family members—including mothers with addictions, serious illness, or learning disabilities, as well as grandparents—have difficulties attending to the physical and psychosocial needs of children when their own health or other needs are great.

A Mother's Story

A single African-American mother in her twenties with a learning disability and chronic asthma has a son who was born premature and has several serious health complications, including asthma and withdrawal from asthma medications. Her mother and stepfather, who were present to assist with the interview, spoke of times when the medical community undermined their daughter's knowledge of the child. When she brought her son to the hospital because he was having an asthma attack, *"the gatekeeper [at the hospital] asked me how I knew my baby was having an asthma attack? I shoved him under her nose and said, 'Blue is not a good color for an African-American baby.'"* The family has also failed to get help because the agencies they utilized competed against one another. Help has come from doctors who truly cared and went the extra mile to help them. *"After we met this one doctor, she immediately turned everything around for [the baby] and got the medications okayed."* Both the mother and the grandparents find it difficult to tend to the child and take him to a doctor because of their rigid work schedules. They are fortunate that the grandfather *"works second shift so [they] can juggle getting [the baby] to the doctor's. . . . it's something as simple as your employer doesn't care that you are a parent."*

System "Meltdown": Agency Competition vs. Coordination of Care

"I realize there are services over there and I'm over here, but I need somebody to talk to who is right here who will know exactly where I'm supposed to go over there. I need somebody in the middle because I don't know which services are going to benefit me the most."

Mother, Allegheny County

Several families described cases in which multiple agencies providing services appeared to compete instead of collaborating in their children's care. One mother hired two nurses to work two different shifts. The nurses did not get along, and when one quit, the mother had to send her sick child away until she could find someone to care for him. In another family, the child was receiving services from two separate agencies. Although the services were not duplicative, one of the agencies released him from its care once it discovered that he was enrolled with another agency. As a result, some of the child's needs went unmet. Provider competition contributes to consumer hopelessness and can lead to despair. What if "competition" were coordinated? What incentives are required to promote greater coordination and collaboration among providers, which could improve delivery of care?

Directions for Change: What Families Want

"We've been asked about problems [in the health care system] before, but nothing ever changes. Will things change now?"

Mother, Allegheny County

The families interviewed demonstrated courage in sharing their stories. They told of painful experiences and described efforts to be resourceful and independent in spite of tremendous needs. Despair and hopelessness are common responses when faced with the "Everest-like mountain" that health care delivery systems have become. What can be done to help families scale this mountain? Families recommended the following directions for change:

- **Improve access.** Families identified several things that would help others identify and use services effectively, such as better information and more transportation. The information should include not only what services are available, but also what rights the families have in obtaining those services, whether they can refuse services, and what responsibility they have in participating. One mother suggested that central locations such as the Welfare Department would be good places to disseminate information, since families that need help have frequent contact there.
- **Enhance coordination.** Families need a liaison to help when multiple agencies are involved. Agencies can take a positive approach to helping families keep track of their needed services and appointments. One mother was pleased to receive reminders about medical checkups for her daughter. Several families also stressed the need for better coordination and collaboration among agencies and less competition.
- **Adopt a family-centered approach to service delivery.** Families recommended that health care agencies pay more attention to the entire family situation, including basic needs and the health of the caregivers as well as those of the children. Mothers noted the need for substance-abuse treatment facilities that can accommodate women with

children. A grandmother talked about the difficulty of caring for her grandchildren when she herself suffers from depression, diabetes, and other health problems. She has trouble giving her grandchildren the full attention doctors suggest that she give. Her recounting of a lack of energy suggests how depression may be a "silent traveler."

- **Instill and assure respect for families.** Perhaps the dominant concern raised by families was how to "get respect" from health care staff and how to eliminate racial and class discrimination. One mother suggested setting up a hotline for reporting discrimination in health care (like the hotline for reporting discrimination in housing). Several mentioned how important it was for the health care provider to listen and to hear the family's story and for the provider interaction to demonstrate respect. Another mother echoed this concern and explained that if staff did not garner trust from the family, including the child, they were unlikely to get families to provide the information they need. The physicians who go the extra mile are the ones who make a difference. While not all health care provision is bad, best practice is far too rare.

CHAPTER FOUR

Barriers and Issues Faced by Local Providers and Program Staff

Ongoing discussions between the project team and the learning collaborative revealed that many local maternal and child health care programs and providers face numerous barriers in their attempts to improve outcomes for mothers with young children. Following the recommendations of learning collaborative members and other community leaders, the project team interviewed 16 local maternal and child health care providers and payers, including county MCOs (providers and payers who were interviewed are listed in Appendix B), to further elucidate these barriers and to uncover possible strategies for overcoming them. In some cases, the barriers and issues described by local providers and program staff were similar in nature to those raised by families in the community (e.g., lack of information). However, the complexities of the issues and the recommendations for resolving them were significantly distinct to warrant additional discussion.

The barriers and issues that emerged from the interviews are divided into two categories: barriers to engaging families, and barriers to coordinating care and integrating services. This chapter concludes with the directions for change recommended by providers and program staff. The project team and the learning collaborative drew on these recommendations, as well as those of families, when formulating the blueprint for action presented in Chapter Seven.

Barriers to Engaging Families at the Local Program Level

"Recruiting staff and enhancing their skills is a major challenge."

Program Staff Member, Allegheny County

Lack of Staff Skills, Numbers, and Types

- Staff must have the skills to establish trusting relationships with families, to apply culturally sensitive approaches that successfully recognize the range of needs that families have, and to address those needs.
- Nurses are generally recognized as an important asset for maternal and child health care programs. Given the current nursing shortage, it is often difficult to hire nurses, more difficult to hire nurses interested in working in community settings, and even more difficult to find nurses who live in the community where the initiative is located.
- Given the high intensity of relationships established in community settings, successful programs need to proactively establish a supportive staff environment that addresses the potential isolation of staff and staff burnout.

Funding Limitations and Licensing Geared to Individual Patient Service

"Current funding mechanisms that reimburse for individual patient (e.g., parent or child) services prevent the provision of integrated service delivery and support to the whole family."

Provider, Allegheny County

- Minimal public investment in prevention and early intervention prevents staff from spending the time required to build relationships with families, to establish trust and rapport, and to meet with families in nontraditional settings (e.g., community sites, families' homes), all of which are considered essential for family engagement.
- There is a lack of funding for "child-friendly facilities" and child care to support parents enrolled in treatment plans.
- The current fee-for-service structure of public funding and its failure to reimburse providers for any of the above activities further exacerbates these problems; building trusting relationships with families is not as difficult when program funding is available.
- Lack of Medicaid funding to support outreach workers who can identify women in need of prenatal care and encourage them to access available services is a particular concern. The current reimbursement structure, which is geared to treatment services within a facility, discourages engagement of families who are more likely to utilize maternal and child health services through home visits or in a community setting. Home-visiting services authorized by the Medicaid MCOs for prenatal and postpartum services are extremely limited.
- Prenatal care services are seldom integrated with behavioral health services, and providers must rely on a different network of health care workers to extend these services through outreach or home-visiting programs.
- Additional licensing regulations that limit the location of service provision discourage family engagement in less-formal community settings and/or in the home.

Factors Impacting Provider/Family Relationships

"The system 'sets families up to fail' when it provides specific services, such as medical care, addiction services, or child-development services without addressing the more basic needs of the family."

Provider, Allegheny County

- Providers and families often do not share the same perception of a child's problem or of his or her need for services. And in cases where providers and families do agree on the need for services, they may each prioritize those needs differently. While the family tends to place highest priority on basic needs (e.g., shelter and food), providers tend to focus on specialized medical care or child-development services.
- Many families are seriously impoverished and therefore lack the resources to either arrange or get to health care appointments. Providers often do not recognize these challenges and mistakenly conclude that the parents are "noncompliant with treatment recommendations."

- Parents tend to have a general distrust of public service providers and thus may not attempt to obtain services for their child from a new provider with whom they have no history.
- Within some families and communities, parents are concerned that any health problem of a child will be viewed as evidence of parental neglect and the child will be removed from the family by child protective services. These concerns exist even in cases where the health concern is clearly not related to neglect.
- Many young children with congenital diseases have related health problems. Parents often spend so much time visiting their pediatrician and other specialists that they have neither the time nor the energy to visit specialty clinics that focus on the child's congenital problems.
- Depression may significantly limit parents' ability to engage with the health care system and to acquire services on behalf of their children, especially in communities where outreach is not well funded.
- Too many providers unrealistically expect that patients will come to them and therefore fail to reach out to those in need of care who may be uncomfortable in professional settings. Far too many pregnant women have no family or support network to engage them in an effective care program. It is also difficult to establish a medical home[1] for families that do not have a stable residence.

Lack of Transportation to Services and Programs

- Travel distances to specialized services or preferred services are a barrier to service provision. Many families cannot afford the cost of public transportation.
- Many providers mentioned issues related to the Medical Assistance Transportation Program (MATP). These include regulations regarding healthy dependents accompanying the family member who is taking a sick child to receive care, reliability, and limitations on what the MATP driver can do to assist passengers.

Barriers to Coordinating Care and Integrating Services at the Local Program Level

Lack of Staff Skills, Numbers, and Types

- Unhelpful and disrespectful staff at key family-serving agencies can hamper effective integration of care.
- Not enough family advocates or care coordinators are available to assist eligible families in obtaining needed and available services.
- Not enough behavioral health specialists are skilled in serving young children (under five years of age) and in addressing problematic relationships between primary caregivers and infants, toddlers, and preschoolers.

---

[1] A medical home provides the patient and her family with a broad spectrum of care over a period of time and coordinates all of the care they receive.

Organizational Silos Created by Funding and Licensing Regulations

- External reimbursement mechanisms create administrative structures within agencies that serve parents and children under separate programs.
- Managed-care behavioral health "carve-outs" prevent linkages between behavioral health and physical health agencies.
- Different regulations, eligibility criteria, and service paradigms within public early-intervention programs (e.g., those for children from birth through two years of age and those for children from three through school age) make transitions difficult for both parents and children. Eligibility limitations with respect to community of residence within the county, age of the children, etc., further complicate service integration.
- Licensing and regulatory limits on the location of service (e.g., service providers can operate only within a licensed facility) and the nature of a service prevent mental health specialists from working with other child-care specialists to provide integrated care. Agencies take a very narrow perspective on what is "allowable" within the reimbursement structure, for fear that an auditor will not permit reimbursement.
- Licensing and regulatory structures discourage the integration of medical information and substance-abuse treatment information for pregnant women.
- Fee-for-service reimbursement sharply limits the amount of time that individual clinicians (e.g., obstetricians, pediatricians, mental health therapists) have to consult with other providers regarding a parent, child, or family or to assist families in connecting with other needed service agencies.
- Confidentiality issues, many of which are related to the new privacy regulations under the Health Insurance Portability and Accountability Act of 1996, are also barriers to coordination of care.

Relationships Among Providers

"We need to create a shared vision of integrated care among leaders of all agencies involved in meeting a family's needs."

Provider, Allegheny County

- The lack of shared responsibility for improving family outcomes creates confusion among providers about their respective roles in serving families, and this confusion can result in gaps in care.
- Professional philosophical differences create barriers to integrated care. In most instances, mental health specialists are unwilling to cross the adult/child line. As a result, an alliance developed with a therapist for one family member (e.g., the mother) cannot be extended to another family member (e.g., a child).
- Child-development professionals and behavioral health specialists do not have a shared paradigm for serving families that will enhance the child's development while addressing the parent's addiction or mental illness.
- Children's pediatricians need to be more fully engaged in family care plans. However, in the view of some child-development providers, pediatricians are often not supportive of early-intervention services, so families choose not to include them.

Lack of Information

- Both families and service providers have difficulty obtaining basic information on services that are available in Allegheny County.
- Lacking sufficient information, providers are frequently unable to tell consumers about other available services.
- Even when providers are aware of other programs that may be appropriate for a family, it is difficult to access pertinent information, such as eligibility requirements and waiting lists, particularly when families move frequently across neighborhoods.

Linkages Across Programs and Services

- There is an urgent need to improve integration within behavioral health and between behavioral health and physical health. Barriers include initial identification of a particular condition (e.g., substance abuse or depression), the individual's ability to recognize the need for treatment, access to treatment, and integrating care across family service providers.
- Lack of coordination of medical care among large hospitals and community services is also an issue. Families often prefer to utilize large, well-respected hospitals (e.g., Magee-Womens Hospital or Children's Hospital of Pittsburgh) for their medical care, and smaller community-based providers (e.g., home visiting services, early-intervention programs) have difficulty coordinating care with hospital-based physicians. Effective communication is particularly challenging among organizations that are a significant distance apart (e.g., the distance between cities such as Clairton and Oakland).
- There are also problems linking and coordinating with WIC, some of which result from the reduced hours and locations of WIC programs across the county.

Directions for Change: What Providers and Program Staff Want

- **Strengthen provider and staff skills.** Providers and program staff need cross-training in cultural competence—how to establish rapport with families; how to recognize and respect families' needs; how to successfully involve families as bona fide collaborators; and how to build upon families' strengths. Child-development professionals need to better understand the parent/child relationship, and behavioral health specialists need to learn how to address the impact of a parent's substance abuse or mental illness on the child's development and how to engage families in appropriate treatment programs, with a particular focus on maternal depression, both during and after pregnancy. Child-care staff need to be able to support children with special-care needs and/or communicable diseases. All staff involved in prenatal services or programs need to be more knowledgeable about nutrition. They should be able to introduce new shopping patterns to families, as well as ways to manage the family food budget. They must also know how to engage social support services in efforts to improve a family's nutrition.
- **Enhance linkages and support relationships among agencies and providers.** A shared vision of integrated care must be created among leaders and across the various levels

of all agencies involved in meeting families' needs. This could be achieved by requiring agencies to jointly define their roles relative both to the family and to each of the agencies that are involved. Establishing a forum in which providers within communities could learn about each other would be useful for supporting the development of more-collaborative relationships and processes. Explicit communication strategies need to be developed among providers for supporting coordinated care for individual families. Stronger linkages between WIC and other family-service programs should be developed and supported.

- **Improve access to information.** The county needs a central clearinghouse of information about available services that is "user-friendly" for both providers and families and that includes information on real-time waiting lists. Although a countywide hot line, operated by the Healthy Start Program and Allegheny County's Department of Health, is available for expectant mothers seeking counseling, assistance, and information on resources and services, many local providers and program staff were not aware of it.

- **Consider new types of reimbursement strategies.** Local providers universally agree that reimbursement for time spent building relationships with families is a prerequisite to effective family engagement.

CHAPTER FIVE

Lessons Learned from Promising National and Local Programs

From a review of the published literature and information on the Internet, the project team identified 12 promising national and local maternal and child health care programs that provide family-centered care and pursue program coordination or integration in a variety of ways (the programs are listed in Appendix C). Members of the project team interviewed representatives of these programs to determine common strategies or practices that might be useful and relevant to local systems-improvement efforts. This chapter summarizes the types of systems and agencies that are typically involved in providing good maternal and child health care, the strategies and practices that model programs employ to engage families, the strategies and practices that model programs pursue to coordinate care or integrate services for families, and the funding streams used to pay for family-engagement and service-coordination activities.

This information was another source upon which the project team and the learning collaborative drew when formulating the blueprint for action presented in Chapter Seven.

Systems and Agencies Involved

"Practitioners and researchers have increasingly embraced the concept that favorable maternal and child health outcomes depend on providing a comprehensive or holistic array of services."

The model programs identified provide a variety of services and coordinate their activities with a range of other service providers. Some programs provide prenatal care and parental education services and coordinate their activities with pediatric or behavioral health care providers. Others integrate behavioral health care and Head Start, while still others focus on care coordination and outreach to identify and engage low-income families.

In general, effective systems and agencies include some combination of the following:

- Obstetrics/gynecology and/or prenatal care
- Pediatric health care (including the Early and Periodic Screening, Diagnosis, and Treatment [EPSDT] mandate)
- Infant/child behavioral health care (mental health services)
- Early intervention (birth to age three)
- Early care and education (generally for children ages three to five)
- Family health care
- Adult behavioral health care (mental health and/or substance-abuse services)

Practitioners and researchers have increasingly embraced the concept that favorable maternal and child health outcomes depend on providing a comprehensive or holistic array of services. While the most effective national programs have overcome a fragmented service delivery system and eased families' access to many (though not necessarily all) of the services they need, none of the programs have been completely successful. Some, for example, offer early intervention and pediatric health services but lack the staff or other resources needed to provide behavioral health services, or they lack collaborative relationships with behavioral health service providers to whom they could refer families. Representatives of all 12 programs mentioned barriers and disappointments in trying to expand the array of services available to their client families. Nevertheless, these programs have made great strides in easing access to care and ensuring that families receive a greater number of services than is typically the case with a fragmented service delivery system.

Strategies and Practices Used to Engage Families

"Families are usually more willing to address behavioral health, chronic disease, and other problems after they have received help with their more immediate needs."

Strengths-Based Treatment Models

Most of the programs interviewed operationalize family-centeredness by employing particular treatment models that focus on families' strengths. These models define the family as the unit of service, placing great emphasis on building strong personal relationships with families and establishing structural activities designed to engage families and ensure that they feel comfortable and respected.

A variety of models exist for engaging and providing services to families. There is no single best model, but most successful service providers select one, provide their staffs with intensive training in it, and fully implement it when working with families. The models often include a curriculum for training staff and protocols for dealing with families. In addition, most of them attend to the needs of both children and parents, usually defining the unit of service as the entire family.

One model, used by several of the programs interviewed, is the Developmental Training and Support Program developed by Victor Bernstein at the University of Chicago (Bernstein, 2002–2003a,b; Bernstein and Campbell, 2001). This model focuses on strengthening the relationship between the parent and the infant or child. Program staff first work on building a strong and trusting relationship with the parent. Central to this process is mutual identification of the family's strengths. Program staff attempt to build on those strengths in developing a mutually agreed-upon service plan with the family, and they support continued family involvement in the implementation and evaluation of the plan. Many of the programs that utilize this model also first address the immediate needs of the family, such as housing, employment, and lack of food. In most cases, addressing these needs involves collaborating with social service providers. Families are usually more willing to address behavioral health, chronic disease, and other problems after they have received help with their more immediate needs.

Strong Relationships with Families and Across Programs

Closely related to the use of specific strengths-based models for engaging families is the development of a strong relationship between program staff and the family. Staff of successful programs spend a great deal of time getting to know families. Many program directors reported that a close bond between service provider and family (especially the parent[s]) is forged over the course of several face-to-face meetings. The establishment of close working relationships with the staff of collaborating programs is equally important, and it also facilitates the engagement of families.

Home-Visiting Programs

Several of the programs interviewed have a home-visiting component. Home visiting can be especially effective in engaging families who are reluctant to seek services at a hospital, clinic, or other facility. It also enables program staff to assess family members' health needs within the context of their living environment (both the home and the neighborhood). In some cases, home visitors are nurses or social workers who provide some services directly and refer families to other providers for other services. In other cases, home visitors are specially trained paraprofessionals (often from within the community being served) who serve as care coordinators, connecting families to service providers and educating them about the range of resources available in the community. The community paraprofessionals are most successful when they reflect the demographics of the population served. One of the programs has home-visiting teams that comprise both a public health nurse and a trained paraprofessional. While the paraprofessional focuses on outreach, educating the family about available services and linking the family to other providers, the nurse provides case management, direct services such as prenatal care and developmental screenings and assessments, and more-detailed medical information.

Location of Programs and Staff

"It is much easier to build relationships with low-income families when services are offered in family-friendly places within their communities."

Staff Person, National Program

Some programs engage families by locating staff in places that low-income families are already frequenting, such as family health clinics, child-care settings, or local health departments. Several of the programs interviewed have found this to be a very effective means of increasing low-income families' utilization of maternal and child health services, echoing much of the recent literature in maternal and child health and child development (Badura, 1999; Center for the Study of Social Policy, 1996; Duggan et al., 2000; National Research Council and the Institute of Medicine, 2000; Schorr, 1997). Program representatives reported that most low-income families prefer to receive services in familiar, family-friendly locations and that this approach eliminates the need for families to travel what are often long distances for services. In some instances, staff from different agencies collocate in a single site, offering a sort of "one-stop-shopping" approach to service provision. Even these programs, however, must refer families to outside providers for certain services.

Use of Lay Staff

Whether they deliver services through home visits or in a family health clinic or other community-based location, some programs find the use of lay staff to be an important means of engaging families. In most cases, lay staff are trained paraprofessionals who serve as outreach workers or care coordinators. Some programs hire former program recipients or others from within the community being served. But other programs have been effective at engaging families and achieving positive health outcomes without the use of lay staff. A few program representatives mentioned that professionals—nurses in particular—often command a higher level of respect from families than lay staff do.

Involvement of Parents

A few programs maintain a family-centered approach in part by involving parents in governance, often as members of advisory boards, such as Head Start policy councils. Most of the programs interviewed, however, do not give families a role in governance but instead allow them to play a major role in developing their own service plans. This typically means that parents decide who will be included on their treatment team and help to determine what the goals of treatment or service use will be. They often invite other family members or friends to be a part of the team. Some of the programs also regularly convene parent discussion or support groups, where parents can learn from and get to know each other and also get better acquainted with program staff. Research suggests that these kinds of activities can be crucial to effective family engagement but that including parents in governance is not essential.

Strategies and Practices Used to Coordinate Care or Integrate Services

Collocating Staff in Community-Based Offices

A number of well-coordinated programs collocate staff in community-based program offices. One model program places adult and child behavioral health specialists in Head Start centers in order to integrate behavioral health services with child-development and nutrition services. Another program places EPSDT outreach workers in local health departments and community health centers that serve low-income families. These workers coordinate EPSDT services with primary care, prenatal care, and other services offered at these locations.

Use of Multidisciplinary Treatment Teams

In many programs, treatment teams include members representing several different service providers who collaborate on a given family's service plan. Members of treatment teams may be substance-abuse counselors, mental health counselors, early-intervention specialists, pediatricians or physicians, and, in some cases, emergency housing staff, food bank representatives, or legal aides. This multidisciplinary approach increases the likelihood that all of a family's needs will be addressed and is an important means of improving a fragmented service delivery system. In some cases, all multidisciplinary staff are employed by the same agency; in others, contractual agreements or memoranda of understanding between agencies ensure that staff from different agencies work together on families' service plans.

Cross-Training of Staff

Some programs encourage greater service coordination by providing cross-training for their staffs. One program that has integrated perinatal, child-development, and child health services provides training in behavioral health for its care coordinators. The training enables the care coordinators, who visit families in their homes, to recognize possible mental health or substance-abuse problems and make proper referrals. In another program, behavioral health specialists provide similar training for child-care and child-development workers, thus strengthening the links between those two systems. Cross-training can also reduce philosophical differences between service providers in different systems, thereby facilitating collaboration between systems (e.g., family health and behavioral health care) and better equipping staff to screen and make proper referrals for problems that fall outside their areas of expertise.

Integrated Information Resources

A few programs have integrated data systems that enable case managers or care coordinators to track individual families and share data across programs. Case managers and care coordinators can determine whether families are eligible for certain services, have a medical home, have received certain services or kept appointments, and so on. Such data systems have been used to develop systematic, streamlined referral and feedback systems across agencies. In addition, many of these systems include data on health outcomes.

Another innovation that has facilitated service coordination in one urban area is a detailed Web-based inventory of all service providers available in the region. Health clinic staff in the area routinely access this database on their computers to identify resources for families. In addition, they can enter data on a family's income and other characteristics to make a preliminary determination of eligibility for specific programs (e.g., Medicaid or WIC).

Personal Relationships

> *". . . effective coordination of services across providers rests as much on personal relationships as on specific structural characteristics."*

In many of the programs, effective coordination of services across providers rests as much on personal relationships as it does on specific structural characteristics. Typically, close ongoing relationships among program directors provided the impetus for coordination, often accompanied or followed by the development of solid relationships between program staff. Unfortunately, such collaborative arrangements tend to be fragile; some program directors described collaborative efforts that suffered or collapsed as a result of leadership changes and staff turnover in partner agencies.

Strong Leadership

Strong leadership is necessary for establishing and maintaining effective partnerships across agencies. Most of the programs interviewed benefited immensely from having at least one strong leader (e.g., an agency director) who took the initiative in contacting other program leaders, developing a plan for service coordination, and securing funding to pay for service coordination activities and other system improvements.

Funding Streams That Pay for Family Engagement and Care Coordination or Service Integration

The project team's interviews suggested that funding family-engagement activities and care-coordination or service-integration efforts is difficult to obtain and requires some creativity, since most funding streams are targeted to direct services. Several programs braid funds from disparate streams to pay for these activities. Others rely primarily on demonstration grants to cover them. Because such funds are usually time-limited, these providers face funding challenges in attempting to sustain their programs. In addition, some programs find that they are better able to fund services for families if they can avoid having to label children (e.g., as being in need of early intervention). Common funding sources include IDEA Part C; EPSDT; Title V, Maternal and Child Health Block Grants; tobacco-settlement funds; state general-revenue funds; Temporary Assistance for Needy Families (TANF); demonstration grants.

Several programs began with demonstration sites and successfully went to scale by convincing their state legislature to appropriate state general-revenue funds to them. These funds are often flexible enough to allow programs to use them to pay for time-consuming family-engagement activities and service-coordination activities. Title V, tobacco-settlement, and TANF block-grant funds have played a similar role for several programs. Being able to bill Medicaid for services also provides a significant source of revenue for program sustainment and expansion, but many providers have noted that Medicaid does little to cover the costs associated with family engagement and service coordination or integration.

CHAPTER SIX

Potential Policy Levers for Enhancing Local Improvement Efforts

Any effort to improve the maternal and child health care system must take into account the full network of government programs and regulations that impact this system. Through programs such as Medicaid and the State Children's Health Insurance Program (SCHIP), government serves as the purchaser of health care services in the public-sector market and can determine the nature of the services it buys through contractual arrangements with managed-care entities. In its capacity as a regulator, government can impose significant legal requirements on health care providers, organizations, and managed-care entities and may set standards regarding the nature and quality of public-sector maternal and child health services.

While there are numerous opportunities for maternal and child health care policy reform at the federal level, the project team focused on state-level policy changes that would be most likely to enhance local improvement efforts. The recommendations presented below are based on the project team's interviews with officials of local Medicaid MCOs, discussions with the learning collaborative, and a review of relevant, publicly available documents. Rather than advocating for sweeping policy change, the recommendations point to concrete leverage points where specific changes can alleviate barriers in some component of the maternal and child health care system. Several of these leverage points will be explored further as part of the community's blueprint for action presented in Chapter Seven. This chapter concludes with some thoughts on broader reforms that could foster additional improvements in maternal and child health care.

While much of the regulatory control for maternal and child health care in the Pittsburgh region rests in the Pennsylvania state capitol of Harrisburg, significant resources are managed locally by leaders who are motivated to improve outcomes for families with young children and who are knowledgeable about providers in the county. Allegheny County's Department of Health and Department of Human Services, as well as the local Medicaid MCOs, play an important role and should be recognized as additional leverage points for improving maternal and child health care programs and services in the region.

Targets for State-Level Policy Reform

On the whole, Medicaid MCO representatives do not view contractual or regulatory burdens as a focal challenge to their efforts for improving maternal and child health care. Those interviewed expressed more concern about their own contractual relationships with maternal and child health care providers, their ability to track performance and outcomes across a range of maternal and child health care services, and their role in encouraging provider coordination and outreach by setting appropriate standards and incentives. The above notwithstanding, four specific targets for state policy reform were identified:

- Information privacy and confidentiality
- Transportation and MATP
- The schism between physical and mental health under Pennsylvania Medicaid
- Coordination between the Pennsylvania DOH and the Pennsylvania DPW

Information Privacy and Confidentiality

The privacy regulations of the Health Insurance Portability and Accountability Act (HIPAA) of 1996, which became effective on April 14, 2003, have spurred intensive efforts by health care providers and plans. In general, the federal rules establish broad privacy rights on behalf of individuals with respect to their own identifiable health information. In addition, HIPAA expressly allows states to enact more-stringent privacy restrictions than those that would apply under federal rules.

Pennsylvania has taken advantage of this flexibility by establishing strict confidentiality standards for both mental health treatment records and drug- and alcohol-abuse treatment records. The Pennsylvania statute broadly restricts the disclosure of mental health records without an individual's written consent, although the designation of a third-party payer is automatically construed as a consent to disclose mental health records to that payer, with the proviso that such disclosure be limited to the information necessary to establish reimbursement claims. The Pennsylvania statute regarding drug and alcohol records is more restrictive and establishes that even with an individual's consent, such records may be disclosed to medical personnel only for purposes of that individual's diagnosis and treatment or to officials for purposes of obtaining benefits due that individual. Only very limited disclosures of drug and alcohol records to an individual's insurance plan are permissible, even with the individual's consent.

Pennsylvania privacy rules are particularly burdensome in the context of public-sector maternal and child health care, where the health care problems and treatment of one family member may directly affect the health status and treatment of other family members. For example, a mother's alcohol problem could have significant ramifications not only for her own physical health, but also for her capacity to care for a child with a chronic illness. Although exchange of treatment information about one or more members of the same family across multiple clinical providers and health plans would greatly enhance efforts to provide integrated family care, Pennsylvania law forbids many of these sorts of disclosures in connection with drug and alcohol treatment and creates substantial barriers to such disclosures in connection with mental health treatment.

The problem is exacerbated by a climate of legal ambiguity in which defensiveness among providers may lead to unduly conservative disclosure practices. These communication problems are not resolvable through the simple expedient of individual consent. Providers inside and outside the mental health treatment system, for example, may have no way of knowing the health status and treatment of other family members—information that would enable them to recognize that a request for disclosure of records might be appropriate. Medicaid MCOs, which seemingly might be in a better position to track and coordinate information-sharing across multiple providers and family members, are in fact unable to do so, in part because of legal restrictions on disclosures to health plans and in part because of the bifurcation of mental and physical health benefits, with treatment provided by different MCOs.

Initial efforts to address the negative impact of the privacy laws on the maternal and child health care system should include legislative and regulatory review of existing privacy rules, focused on revising those rules to facilitate communication between mental health providers, drug- and alcohol-treatment providers, and others in the health care system. Moreover, the rules should ideally permit some communication between providers for different members of the same family, at least with the written consent of the adults. Finally, the rules should better accommodate the reality that health-plan staff may be in the best position to track information across multiple providers and family members and might therefore serve a coordinating function that goes beyond claims reimbursement. At the very least, the state needs to clarify ambiguities in its privacy rules and to educate health care stakeholders regarding the scope of appropriate disclosures in the context of family-centered, multidisciplinary, cross-institutional maternal and child health care.

Transportation and MATP

The best maternal and child health care system in the world is effective only if consumers can readily gain access to it. Community-based outreach and case management aside, many sorts of maternal and child services require travel to physicians' offices, hospitals, or other types of health care facilities. For a mother who depends on public transportation, has multiple children and limited social supports, and a job with limited flexibility for absence, transportation to and from health care appointments can be a significant impediment to obtaining good care. In recognition of this problem, Pennsylvania enacted the Medical Assistance Transportation Program (MATP), a state initiative that "administers the provision of non-emergency medical transportation services to Medical Assistance [e.g., Medicaid] clients who cannot meet their own transportation needs" (Pennsylvania Office of Social Programs, n.d.).

MATP is organized as a state-county partnership in which Pennsylvania counties (including Allegheny County) receive funding from the state to establish their own MATPs. To receive state funding, counties must operate their MATPs pursuant to Pennsylvania regulations that establish eligibility criteria for access to MATP services, prevent counties from imposing any additional eligibility requirements, and compel counties to perform (auditable) eligibility determinations. Within these guidelines, however, the counties (and their designated contractors) have significant latitude in how they actually operate their MATPs. The counties develop their own procedures for determining MATP eligibility and exercise subjective judgment when evaluating (and documenting) need for MATP services. Counties have the discretion to reduce or terminate MATP services to individual clients, based on a professional judgment that services are no longer needed or that a client's "uncooperative behavior or misuse of services" warrants termination. The counties are permitted, but not required, to pay transportation costs for escorts (i.e., noneligible persons who accompany eligible clients to needed medical services). Apart from a provision concerning priority scheduling in peak periods of demand, Pennsylvania regulations do not specify or mandate particular benefits in connection with county MATPs.

Access to MATPs is complicated by the fact that each county operates its own transportation program. Particularly in rural counties, a need for maternal and child health services may require clients to cross county lines—something that is reportedly difficult to accomplish using MATP transportation. More generally, Pennsylvania imposes no single standard on the counties with regard to allowing mothers to bring their dependent children onto MATP transportation, even though the inability to do so can significantly restrict mothers' access to services. Although state rules do provide beneficiaries with a right to appeal adverse MATP decisions, that appeal right could have limited value for many low-income mothers, whose primary concern is to obtain needed health care services and for whom arranging transportation to a "fair hearing" may be as problematic as arranging transportation to a physician's office.

Clearly, MATP offers a promising target for state-level policy reform. Although the state/county partnership structure of MATP may be a reasonable way to deliver transportation services, the state should set standards that allow mothers to bring their dependent children on MATP transportation, provide a clear mandate to counties regarding MATP transportation across county lines, and establish more-specific and uniform guidelines regarding the determination of need for MATP services.

Schism Between Physical and Mental Health Under Pennsylvania Medicaid

One of the most striking features of the public-sector health care system in Pennsylvania (and in Allegheny County) is the division between physical health MCOs and providers and behavioral health MCOs and providers, formalized by the state's Medicaid waiver, which establishes separate contractual mechanisms for each system (Commonwealth of Pennsylvania, Department of Public Welfare, 1997). The state contracts directly with three MCOs to manage Medicaid physical health benefits in Southwest Pennsylvania, but it contracts with county governments to manage behavioral health benefits. In turn, the counties (including Allegheny County) subcontract with a fourth MCO that administers the behavioral health carve-out under Medicaid. In the context of providing care for mothers and children, the result has been to make cross-system collaboration and information-sharing difficult.

The separation between physical and behavioral health care under Medicaid offers a good target for maternal and child health policy reform in Pennsylvania. As mentioned above, state privacy rules reinforce the division between physical and behavioral health care providers in ways that can make coordination of maternal and child health care difficult to achieve. Another problem that arises under the current system involves the division of responsibility between Medicaid MCOs. For example, while a behavioral MCO carries responsibility for managing most aspects of behavioral health services, the physical MCOs retain responsibility for managing pharmacy benefits, including psychotropic drugs. As a result, the physical MCOs are compelled to make determinations about the appropriateness of prescriptions in the absence of information about behavioral health care (which the behavioral MCO is reportedly not entitled to share).

MCOs and providers on both sides of the division should be engaged in appropriate information-sharing and tracking of maternal and child health services, in order to provide effective care. State policy should support this kind of collaboration by formally recognizing the need for partnership across physical and behavioral health care systems and between physical and behavioral health MCOs. Accordingly, state laws and state Medicaid contracts not only should facilitate related communications and information-sharing, but should, in fact, require them.

Coordination Between Pennsylvania DOH and Pennsylvania DPW

The maternal and child health care system in Allegheny County (and in Pennsylvania more generally) is characterized by silos of different providers and organizations that address specific aspects of maternal and child health care, with only limited coordination across them. Divisions between physical and behavioral health, adult and pediatric services, and hospital-based services and primary care create barriers to the integration of maternal and child health care services.

Enhanced collaboration between state government agencies is an important first step toward improving the maternal and child health system. One of the major potential collaborations in state government would be between Pennsylvania DOH and Pennsylvania DPW.

Pennsylvania DPW provides administrative oversight for a number of different state-level social service and public-assistance programs, including those generally related to children, families, mental health, developmental disability, welfare, and Medicaid (Commonwealth of Pennsylvania, Department of Public Welfare, n.d.). With respect to maternal and child health, DPW's most vital function is its oversight of Medicaid, as exercised through its Office of Medical Assistance Programs. In that capacity, DPW contracts with MCOs to provide maternal and child health benefits to mothers and children and tracks Medicaid performance on a variety of measures.

By contrast, Pennsylvania DOH is a public-health agency. DOH executes a number of health-related administrative functions for the state, including health needs assessment, assuring access to quality care, promoting health and preventing disease, and engaging in health policy development and health planning activities (Department of Health, Background Information). One of the important aspects of DOH's role as a public health agency is its collection of health care data across the state through its Bureau of Health Statistics and Research. Data collected by DOH serve "to assist in evaluating the health status of Pennsylvania residents, and the quality . . . of health services [throughout the state]" (Health: Bureau of Health Statistics and Research, n.d.). Thus, DOH is broadly involved in prevention measures and health care quality assessment, as supported by statewide data collection and analysis—all functions that are highly relevant to maternal and child health care.

DOH also has a Bureau of Community Health Systems, which operates a network of six medical districts and 57 health centers and serves as the implementation arm for the department's public-health programs. The district offices provide coordination, consultative, and administrative support to the health centers, including communicable-disease reporting and investigation, epidemiology, information and referral, chronic-disease prevention and intervention programs, communicable-disease clinical services, family health programs, and environmental health services. In addition, health centers engage in community health-assessment and quality-assurance activities and provide other public health services, including community integration and outreach programs, to promote healthy behaviors. The bureau oversees the coordination of similar programs with four municipal and six county health departments, including the Allegheny County Department of Health.

Several MCOs and members of the learning collaborative commented that Pennsylvania DPW and DOH have not yet fulfilled their potential for synergy. Several anecdotal examples were offered of DOH health-reporting requirements (e.g., in connection with lead exposure) that DPW reportedly undermined through changes in its own forms and regulations, thus making it impossible for DOH to carry out some aspects of its data-collection mission. It has been suggested that the WIC program administered by DOH offers a logical entry point into the maternal and child health system and could assist other maternal and child health programs (particularly Medicaid under DPW) by sharing elements of its enrollment data (Cavanaugh, Lippit, and Moyo, 2000). WIC's reluctance to do so illustrates a significant communication gap between DPW and DOH and highlights the fact that the two departments have engaged in only limited collaboration in the making of health policy.

To their credit, both departments have acknowledged the importance of interdepartmental initiatives in future efforts to improve the health care system in Pennsylvania (Pennsylvania Department of Health, 2001). With regard to maternal and child health care, the two departments should ideally be in consultation on areas where their functions overlap (e.g., data collection and quality assessment), while capitalizing on areas of complementary strength (e.g., DOH's focus on public-health infrastructure and prevention and DPW's on the direct delivery of services). Recent steps toward reform made by policymakers in Harrisburg suggest that these sorts of departmental changes may be in the offing.

Key recommendations for state-level policy reform are summarized in Table 6.1.

Table 6.1
Key Recommendations for State-Level Policy Reform

Information privacy and confidentiality	Pennsylvania state policymakers to revise state privacy laws to facilitate treatment communications between mental health/substance-abuse-treatment providers and other providers, as well as between providers for different family members
Transportation and MATP	Educate Pennsylvania state policymakers to set standards that guarantee public transportation for families seeking access to maternal and child health care through MATP services
Schism between physical and mental health under Pennsylvania Medicaid	Pennsylvania state policymakers to require that state laws and state Medicaid contracts mandate communication and information-sharing regarding maternal and child health care services across physical and behavioral health care systems and between physical and behavioral health MCOs
	State and local policymakers to build mechanisms for collaboration among state and local departments that share responsibility for children, mothers, and families in order to simplify procedures regarding families' access to benefits and services and to reduce the burden of legal/ admin-istrative requirements and regulations on providers

Toward Broader Policy Reform

Beyond these specific prescriptions for state maternal and child health policy reform, several more-general policy themes emerged during the interviews and discussions with the learning collaborative. These themes are summarized below:

- Maternal and child health care providers are substantially overburdened by legal and administrative requirements related to licensing laws, Medicaid and public-health regulations, managed-care contractual provisions, etc. Administrative paperwork and reporting cut dramatically into time spent in direct patient contact. In recognition of this problem, policymakers in Harrisburg are reviewing the regulatory burdens carried by public-sector health care providers, with an eye toward reducing those burdens where possible.

- Medicaid reimbursement policies in Pennsylvania significantly favor medical specialists over primary care providers (reimbursement policies reportedly differ from state to state). This could create a disincentive to the provision of maternal and child primary care under Medicaid. A more systematic investigation of the impact of state regulations and reimbursement policies on providers is an appropriate future task.
- Many of the government programs, provider organizations, and health plans that comprise the maternal and child health care system engage in some kind of data collection, with regard to either service utilization or health outcomes. Clinical and health-status data are vital to any community-based effort to improve maternal and child health care, since such information is needed to show that particular interventions or reforms result in measurable improvement in outcomes. But data collection presents two core challenges: (1) determining what kinds of information are needed to support maternal and child health care quality-improvement efforts and who should collect it, and (2) eliminating redundancy and minimizing the burdens of collection, while ensuring data access for appropriate users. State policymakers have an important role to play in facilitating community-based maternal and child health care data collection, through streamlining reporting processes, eliminating duplicative and conflicting regulatory requirements, and partnering with regional maternal and child health care quality-assessment efforts.
- Interdepartmental collaborations in Pennsylvania might offer unrealized synergies, connected either to the maternal and child health care system or to other sorts of social programs that support low-income mothers and children. For example, recent efforts by DPW and the Pennsylvania Department of Insurance to adopt joint enrollment forms for Medicaid and SCHIP should simplify the application process for parents who are unfamiliar with the distinctions between the two programs (Pennsylvania Children's Health Insurance Program, 2001). Similarly, the Pennsylvania executive branch is now exploring ways to build greater coordination between its departments, for example, by the establishment of a Children and Family Cabinet consisting of the leadership of several departments with shared responsibility for children and families. These kinds of reforms show promise that Pennsylvania agencies and programs can find new, low-cost ways to facilitate their collective missions.
- Recognizing that the financial incentives incorporated in both regulations and contractual relationships among government, MCOs, and providers ultimately determine the kinds of maternal and child health services the system actually offers, financial incentives should be structured to ensure the provision of needed categories of service, and performance-based compensation should be used to drive quality improvement. Pennsylvania DPW is already considering ways to implement performance-based financial incentives for the state's Medicaid MCOs, and such incentives might also be fielded in many other parts of the maternal and child health care system (e.g., between MCOs and provider organizations or between provider organizations and their employees).

CHAPTER SEVEN

A Blueprint for Community Action

Community stakeholders seeking to improve the Pittsburgh region's maternal and child health care system face a number of daunting challenges that defy any single program or policy prescription. As the findings of this report illustrate, maternal and child health care involves a vast array of programs and services; numerous and multifaceted relationships among government agencies, MCOs, and health care providers; and a complex patchwork of federal, state, and local policies that to varying degrees help shape the nature and quality of public-sector maternal and child health care services. Caught in this system are the consumers of health care services, who must bear the impact of its inefficiencies and inadequacies while simultaneously meeting their other basic life needs.

Clearly, any effort to confront the multiple issues that impact the overall maternal and child health care system will require a vision of tremendous breadth and power that originates from the community's own needs, values, and goals. This vision, in turn, must inform an ongoing change strategy that reflects the broad array of critical factors and influences that determine the health of individuals, families, and communities. These factors range from individual behaviors and the overall community environment to specific practices, programs, and policies that affect the way health care is delivered. To be achievable and sustainable over the long term, the strategy must drive an action plan that encompasses significant and widespread changes in consciousness and practice; unprecedented cooperation among federal, state, and local governments and between and among the different departments and agencies within these organizations; new types of public-private partnerships to leverage existing infrastructure supports; resources to reduce disparities in access and quality of care; and public education and engagement campaigns that attempt to change public attitudes and standards, educate community residents, and support community-based interventions.

Vision

Members of the Pittsburgh region's learning collaborative have identified the following key components of their shared vision for achieving an outstanding local maternal and child health care system:

- Promote healthy lifestyles and positive health outcomes
- Reduce preventable disease and environmental health risks
- Eliminate health disparities
- Ensure access to quality care for young children, mothers, and families

Ideally, such a system will have the following characteristics:

- An established medical or social service home or homes for each family in the community and/or each mother and her child(ren)
- A family-centered, culturally competent approach to care, in which providers address the needs of and draw on the strengths of the entire family being served
- Integrated/holistic services, with service providers working closely together, addressing all aspects of a family's health and social needs that impact the at-risk child
- A high-quality maternal and child health care workforce, well trained in the principles of family-centeredness, cultural competence, and integrated/holistic care
- Families well educated about available programs and resources and about healthy behaviors (e.g., proper nutrition, the importance of prenatal care, smoking cessation, reducing environmental health risks) and empowered to demand high-quality maternal and child health care
- Effective leadership at the state and county levels, with clear lines of authority and accountability for performance

Strategy

To achieve this vision, a RAND–University of Pittsburgh project team, in collaboration with local leaders of the maternal and child health care system, will:

- Expand and further engage the existing local maternal and child health care stakeholders' learning collaborative to form a *leadership collaborative* with the power and authority to establish priorities, mobilize available resources, guide and support community-based quality-improvement interventions, measure outcomes, and advocate for change in policy, financing, and practice at the state and local levels
- Advance a *family-centered approach* to maternal and child health care that (1) establishes a medical or social service home or homes for each family in the community and/or each mother and her child(ren); (2) recognizes a family's strengths while seeking to understand and meet its basic and other health care needs; and (3) is nurtured in an environment of cultural competency and trusting, respectful relationships
- Promote effective *coordination and integration of care and outreach*, particularly between and among physical health care, behavioral health care, environmental health programs, and social-support services
- Develop plans to establish *countywide integrated data systems* that (1) provide useful information on available services and resources for families, (2) support practitioners' efforts to coordinate care and track a family's progress across agencies and programs, (3) enable agencies to monitor service utilization and performance across individual programs, and (4) support health plans in developing flexible, performance-based payment structures that ensure provision of needed services and drive quality-improvement efforts at the provider and practitioner levels

Each of these strategies will focus on the community's key priority areas:

- Prenatal care
- Family behavioral health
- Nutrition
- Chronic illness and special-care needs

Action Plan

Outlined below is a complete set of action steps for the Pittsburgh region that should be implemented by specific stakeholder groups at various levels of the maternal and child health care system, with the local stakeholders' leadership collaborative serving as the organizing entity.

- At the *state/local policy level*, the action plan will expand the engagement of community stakeholders; improve the dissemination of information on maternal and child health care programs, services, and resources; build the community's capacity to monitor health outcomes for provider accountability and quality improvement; target specific areas for regulatory, licensing, and other policy reform; and enhance advocacy for improving maternal and child health care.
- At the *payer/plan* level, the action plan will promote the design of financial and other incentives that will ensure provision of needed services and drive quality-improvement efforts at the provider and practitioner levels.
- At the *agency/program/provider* level, the action plan will establish new types of training, strategies, and practice that will result in increased family engagement and care coordination.

Each of these steps is described in detail below, with specific actions designated across key players in the maternal and child health care system in order to establish clear lines of accountability for their implementation. The action steps have been developed based on the recommendations of families in the community and local providers and program staff (Chapters Three and Four), the experiences of model national and local programs (Chapter Five), and the state-level policy levers identified in Chapter Six.

While some components of the plan clearly are resource- and time-intensive (e.g., development of mechanisms for countywide integrated data collection, analysis, and dissemination of maternal and child health care outcomes), others should be relatively simple to implement (e.g., enhancing the visibility and use of the existing countywide hotline for expectant mothers). In an ideal world, all components of the plan would be implemented simultaneously, but various components could be prioritized and implemented according to level of greatest perceived need, available resources, etc.

Actions for State and Local Policy Leaders

- Formalize and expand the local stakeholders' leadership collaborative with a mandate to improve maternal and child health care service delivery and outcomes in the Pittsburgh region
  - Convene an independent entity that includes leaders of Allegheny County's Department of Health and Department of Human Services
  - Ensure continued involvement of the primary payers of maternal and child health care services in the Pittsburgh region
  - Enhance family participation by facilitating and supporting family representatives to develop a bona fide role in the leadership collaborative
  - Strengthen linkages with state policymakers in the Pennsylvania DOH and Pennsylvania DPW and include them as members of the leadership collaborative
- Assign the leadership collaborative oversight responsibility for the implementation of the following specific actions:
  - Advocate for needed policy reform
    - Build mechanisms for collaboration among state and local departments that share responsibility for children, mothers, and families in order to simplify procedures regarding families' access to benefits and service and to reduce the burden of legal and administrative requirements and regulations on providers
    - Educate state policymakers to guarantee public transportation for families seeking access to maternal and child health care through MATP services
    - Require state laws and Medicaid contracts to mandate communication and information-sharing regarding maternal and child health care services across the physical and behavioral health care systems and between physical and behavioral health MCOs
    - Revise state privacy laws to facilitate treatment communication between mental health and substance-abuse treatment providers and other providers and to permit communication among providers for different members of the same family
    - Change licensing laws that make it difficult to operate programs for families in a single setting
    - In all cases, establish appropriate performance measures to ensure that the policy changes are effective
  - Plan, implement, and track the progress of a health-promotion campaign that educates families and consumers about how to demand quality service
  - Improve information dissemination on maternal and child health care services and related resources (e.g., behavioral health, housing, child care) for both families and providers
    - Create "user-friendly" communication mechanisms to give families and providers the information they need
    - Enhance the visibility and use of the countywide hotline for expectant mothers seeking counseling, assistance, and information
    - Develop maternal and child health care interest groups that will enable providers within and across communities to learn about each other

– Develop mechanisms for countywide integrated data collection, analysis, and dissemination of maternal and child health care outcomes

- Work with Pennsylvania DOH and DPW and Medicaid plans to explore viable options for integrating information systems that track key measures of health and health disparities
- Construct locally relevant measures of maternal and child health care service utilization and outcomes to support quality-improvement efforts, particularly those designed to reduce health care disparities for low-income mothers and children
- Periodically publish an objective, comprehensive, and useful report card on the status of the Pittsburgh region's maternal and child health care
- Develop measures of the leadership collaborative's success in effecting change

– Provide a local forum through which agency directors, program leaders, and families can create a shared vision of family-centered, coordinated care and develop training and improvement strategies for achieving that vision

– Encourage and support the development of proven models of family-centered, coordinated care (e.g., Starting Early Starting Smart Programs, Early Head Start, Nurse Family Partnerships) that involve strategic partnerships across payers/plans, agencies/programs, and families

Actions for Payers/Plans

- Expand the capacity of local health plans to drive quality improvement by shifting reimbursement incentives to encourage:
  - Efforts by providers to build trusting relationships with families and to extend the social network for making valid and reliable referrals
  - Implementation of family-bundled services
  - Coordinated, longitudinal primary care services
  - More outreach, engagement activities, and prenatal/infant home-based services with documented positive outcomes
  - Care coordinators focused on maternal and child health care across agencies and services (e.g., the special-needs coordinators used by physical health Medicaid MCOs)
  - More culturally relevant caregiver and family behavioral health services, infant and toddler mental health services, and caregiver/infant relationship support services
  - Health care benefits and services for grandparents and/or other family members who are nonparental primary caregivers

- Work with the leadership collaborative and community-based systems-improvement demonstration teams on the development of flexible, performance-based payment structures that reward teams for:
  - Conducting cross-training of staff in the family-strengths-based approach that results in demonstrable improvement
  - Preparing families and staff for the empowered-family role
  - Developing strategic partnerships designed to implement evidence-based interventions that address the needs of multiple family members in an integrated fashion
  - Adopting best clinical practices at the community level

– Extending services beyond small numbers of participants enrolled in special programs to the patient population at large

Actions for Agencies/Programs/Providers

- Work with the leadership collaborative and community-based quality-improvement demonstration teams to:
  - Refocus cross-organizational culture on the family (e.g., the mother, her children, and other significant caregivers), rather than the individual patient, as the unit of care
  - Increase family engagement through involvement in program governance (e.g., as members of advisory boards) and sharing the responsibility for developing their individual service plans
  - Endorse flexibility and risk-taking in meeting families' needs, rather than simply "following the rules"
  - Develop concrete plans for standardized training and service coordination across organizations, with explicit linkages to the family's medical home
  - Design data systems and financing mechanisms that will support such plans
  - Identify a project team in each agency to represent and champion the leadership collaborative in-house
  - Build a family-strengths-based approach to care:
    - Respecting, listening, and responding to families
    - Understanding the family's perspective
    - Seeking family input and mutually identifying its basic needs (e.g., housing, food, transportation, etc.)
    - Helping families to meet those needs by building on their strengths
  - Develop strong, trusting relationships between staff and families
  - Strengthen relationships between the parent/caregiver and the infant or child
  - Improve cultural competency, professional objectivity, and the ability to work outside traditional boundaries and across diverse community settings
  - Enhance specific provider skills in targeted areas, such as infants' social and emotional development, proper nutrition, and working with children with special needs
- Educate providers and practitioners across disciplines and throughout their careers (with a particular emphasis on student programs for physicians and nurses); offer continual reinforcement and support, possibly through state accreditation programs; and track the results of cross-training to document its effectiveness
- Engage family members in identifying and implementing specific strategies that will be effective in working with other families across different cultures and subcultures

Toward a Model Maternal and Child Health Care System in the Pittsburgh Region

To bring this blueprint for action to life, between January 2004 and December 2005, the project team will conduct a policy- and practice-improvement demonstration in the Pittsburgh region that will operate under the direction of an expanded stakeholders' leadership collaborative. The goal of the demonstration is to begin building a model maternal and child health care system that will lead to improved health care for mothers and children from birth to five years of age in the region. The demonstration will have several unique characteristics. First, it will operate on two complementary levels: policy (from the top down) and practice (from the bottom up). Second, it will involve a wide range of key community stakeholders and community-based partnerships in the actual conduct of the work. Third, it will integrate, rather than replicate, existing services and programs. And fourth, it will build important linkages across physical health, behavioral health, environmental health, and other related social-support services.

At the *policy level*, the project team will:

- Organize two policy working groups comprising relevant local stakeholders to develop plans for (1) integrated countywide data collection, analysis, and dissemination of information on maternal and child health care service utilization and outcomes; and (2) flexible, performance-based payment mechanisms that reward quality improvement. These groups will review similar efforts undertaken by other counties and regions, including reports in the literature; assess regulatory, practical, and financial barriers to successful implementation; and identify viable options and strategies for pilot testing of new data-collection and payment mechanisms.
- Support the leadership collaborative in its efforts to tailor and implement proposed policy changes in the Pittsburgh region.

At the *practice level*, the project team will:

- Create and support at least two community-based practice-improvement teams that will (1) involve strategic partnerships among local payers/plans, programs, and families in previously designated high-risk communities; (2) gather baseline information on specific indicators related to the key priority areas of prenatal care, nutrition, behavioral health, and chronic-illness and special-care needs, with linkages to environmental health; (3) adopt and test proven processes and practices for increasing family engagement and care coordination in accordance with the plan-act-study-do rapid-cycle quality-improvement model; and (4) develop data systems and financing mechanisms to support these practice improvements. The project team will provide technical assistance to the practice-improvement teams as they formulate strategic plans that include (1) cross-training of staff in the family-strengths-based model, cultural competency, etc.; (2) clinical and administrative practice improvements; (3) agreed-upon measurement processes and instruments for monitoring outcomes and ensuring provider accountability; (4) financing mechanisms that support quality improvement; and (5) strategies for achieving sustainability and diffusion.
- Monitor and evaluate the progress of the community-based practice-improvement teams. The evaluation will be based on process and outcomes data provided by the individual teams, as well as changes on key indicators of family engagement and care coordination measured first at baseline and then at the completion of the action plans.

- Synthesize the information from the evaluation into a community report card documenting the progress of the community-based practice-improvement teams.
- Develop a countywide plan for the sustainability and diffusion of quality-improvement strategies that are shown to enhance maternal and child health care.

The primary outcomes of this policy- and practice-improvement demonstration will be:

- A local leadership collaborative structure and process for improving policy and practice components of the maternal and child health care system that have been identified as priorities by community stakeholders.
- Communitywide plans for (1) integrated data collection, analysis, and dissemination of information on maternal and child health care service utilization and outcomes; and (2) flexible, performance-based payment mechanisms. Both plans will incorporate strategies for overcoming anticipated barriers.
- Community-based practice-improvement teams that have demonstrated and documented their success.
- Mechanisms that will enable the sustainability and diffusion of the improvement process.

Generalizability to Other Communities

Recognizing that communities differ markedly with respect to their history, demographics, economy, and governance, it is uncertain whether the community-based collaborative process undertaken in the Pittsburgh region for improving maternal and child health care could take hold as effectively in other areas. Certainly, to a large degree, the success of this process locally will be attributable to the historical importance of the family in the community, the energy and cohesiveness of community leadership, and the ability to mobilize significant resources to support visionary change

At the same time, the idea of creating healthy communities is gaining momentum across cities and counties both in the United States and around the world. Although in most cases these communities have identified goals and pursued action plans related to issues other than maternal and child health care, they share many of the same characteristics with the Pittsburgh region, including a common vision, a willingness to work collaboratively, a free flow of information among all major stakeholders, and clear opportunities for improvement. In this sense, Pittsburgh's experience in designing a community blueprint for action could prove useful to a range of communities regardless of the goals they are pursuing.

For those seeking improvement in maternal and child health care in particular, or in service delivery to families in poverty more generally, many of the best practices, barriers, and potential solutions discussed in this report could serve as a basis for developing a community-based collaborative approach designed specifically to address their communities' needs.

Members of the Learning Collaborative

Carmen Anderson
Program Officer for Children, Youth and Families
The Heinz Endowments

Michael Blackwood
President and CEO
Gateway Health Plan

Aurelia Carter
Disability Agenda Issue Organizer
Consumer Health Coalition

Marc Cherna
Director
Allegheny County Department of Human Services

Bob Cicco
President
PA American Academy of Pediatrics

Bruce Dixon
Director
Allegheny County Health Department

Anne Docimo
Vice President of Medical Affairs
UPMC Health Plan

Donald Fischer
Medical Director
Highmark Blue Cross and Blue Shield

Irene Frederick
Consultant in Obstetrics and Gynecology
East Liberty Family Health Care Center;
Consultant in Obstetrics and Gynecology Faculty for Family Medicine Residency, Ob/Gyn
UPMC-Shadyside Family Medicine Residency Program

Bernard D. Goldstein
Dean, Graduate School of Public Health
University of Pittsburgh

Elaine Harris-Fulton
Parent Advocate
Wilkinsburg Family Support Center

Charles LaVallee
Executive Director
The Western Pennsylvania Caring Foundation for Children

John Lovelace
Chief Program Officer
Community Care Behavioral Health Organization

Eugenia Mosby
Children's Enrollment Specialist
Consumer Health Coalition

Jeffrey Palmer
CEO
Coordinated Care Network
Member
Allegheny County Children's Cabinet

Wilford Payne
Executive Director of Primary Care Services
Healthy Start, Inc.

Reverend Ron Peters
Pittsburgh Theological Seminary

Margaret Petruska
Director for Children, Youth and Families
The Heinz Endowments

Father Regis Ryan
Director
STO-ROX Focus on Renewal

Walt Smith
Executive Director
Family Resources

Elizabeth Stork
Former Director of Community Impact Strategy, Health, Seniors, and Foundation Relations
United Way of Allegheny County

Sheila Ward
Medical Director
Three Rivers Health Plan

Rachel Anne Wilson
Director
Children's Cabinet
Allegheny County Department of Human Services

Local Providers and Payers Interviewed

Alliance for Infants and Toddlers, Inc.
The Hough Building
2801 Custer Avenue
Pittsburgh, PA 15227

Center for Children and Families
Western Psychiatric Institute and Clinic
3811 O'Hara Street
Pittsburgh, PA 15213

Community Care Behavioral Health Organization
One Chatham Center
Suite 700, 112 Washington Place
Pittsburgh, PA 15219

Down's Syndrome Center
Children's Hospital of Pittsburgh
3420 Fifth Avenue
Pittsburgh, PA 15213

East Liberty Family Health Care Center
6023 Harvard Street
Pittsburgh, PA 15206

Family Foundations/Early Head Start Program
224 Helen Street
McKees Rocks, PA 15136

Family Services of Western Pennsylvania
6401 Penn Avenue, Second Floor
Pittsburgh, PA 15206

Gateway Health Plan
Two Chatham Center
Suite 500
Pittsburgh, PA 15219

Greater Pittsburgh Community Food Bank
1 North Linden
Duquesne, PA 15110

Healthy Beginnings Plus
Shadyside Hospital
Family Health Center
5215 Centre Avenue
Pittsburgh, PA 15232

Magee at Clairton Health Center
559 Miller Avenue
Clairton, PA 15025

Maternal and Child Health Program
Allegheny County Health Department
907 West Street
Pittsburgh, PA 15221

Mercy Behavioral Health
Pittsburgh Mercy Health System
1200 Reedsdale Street
Pittsburgh, PA 15233

Perinatal Addiction Center
5916 Penn Avenue
Pittsburgh, PA 15206

Three Rivers Health Plans, Inc.
300 Oxford Drive
Monroeville, PA 15146

UPMC Health Plan
One Chatham Center
112 Washington Place
Pittsburgh, PA 15219

Model National and Local Programs Interviewed

Casey Family Partners: Spokane (Starting Early Starting Smart Program)
613 South Washington
Spokane, WA 99204

Comprehensive Health Investment Project of Virginia
701 East Franklin Street
Suite 502
Richmond, VA 23219

F.O.R. Families Program (Follow-Up, Outreach, and Referral)
Bureau of Family and Community Health
250 Washington Street, Fifth Floor
Boston, MA 02108

Great Expectations Foundation
Healthy Start Program
2020 Jackson Avenue
Suite 100
New Orleans, LA 70113

Health Start Program
Office of Women and Children's Health
2927 North 35th Street
Suite 300
Phoenix, AZ 85017

Healthy Start, Inc.
400 North Lexington Ave.
Pittsburgh, PA 15208

Help Me Grow
Ohio Department of Health
Bureau of Early Intervention Services
246 North High Street
Columbus, OH 43216-0118

Miami's Families (Starting Early Starting Smart Program)
University of Miami
P.O. Box 016960
M-808
Miami, FL 33101

New Wish (Starting Early Starting Smart Program)
Nevada Division of Child and Family Services
6171 West Charleston Ave.
Building 16
Las Vegas, NV 89146

North Carolina Health Check Program
North Carolina Department of Health and Human Services
Division of Women's and Children's Health
Health Check
1330 St. Mary's Street
Raleigh, NC 27626

Nurse-Family Partnership Program
National Center for Children, Families, and Communities
1825 Marion Street
Denver, CO 80218

Starting Early to Link Enhanced Comprehensive Treatment Teams
    (SELECTT—Starting Early Starting Smart Program)
University of New Mexico Health Sciences Center
School of Medicine and University Hospital
317 Commercial Street, NE
Suite 100
Albuquerque, NM 87102

References

Aligne, C. A., and J. J. Stoddard (1997). "Tobacco and Children: An Economic Evaluation of the Medical Effects of Parental Smoking," *Archives of Pediatric and Adolescent Medicine,* Vol. 151, No. 7, pp. 648–653.

Allegheny County Health Department (n.d.). On-line Health Beat, http://www.county.allegheny.pa.us/achd/hbeat/0006/hbeat.asp.

Allegheny County Health Department (n.d.). On-line Health Reports, http://www.county.allegheny.pa.us/achd/reports/child20/index.asp.

Allegheny County Health Department (1999, 2000a). Allegheny County Birth Statistics.

Allegheny County Health Department (2000b). *Period of Risks Report.*

Allegheny County Health Department (2003). *Allegheny County Data Bay Navigate Trend Report by Discharges.*

Annie E. Casey Foundation (1999). *The Right Start: Conditions of Babies and Their Families in America's Largest Cities—A Kids Count Special Report,* Baltimore, MD: Annie E. Casey Foundation.

Badura, M. (1999). "The Healthy Start Program: Mobilizing to Reduce Infant Mortality and Morbidity," *Journal of Pediatric Nursing,* Vol. 14, No. 4.

Bernstein, V. (2002–2003a). "Standing Firm Against the Forces of Risk: Supporting Home Visiting and Early Intervention Workers Through Reflective Supervision." *Newsletter of the Infant Mental Health Promotion Project,* Vol. 35, Winter.

Bernstein, V. (2002–2003b). "Strengthening Families Through Strengthening Relationships: Supporting the Parent-Child Relationship Through Home Visiting," *Newsletter of the Infant Mental Health Promotion Project,* Vol. 35, Winter.

Bernstein, V., and S. Campbell (2001). "Caring for the Caregivers: Supporting the Well-Being of At-Risk Parents and Children Through Supporting the Well-Being of the Programs That Serve Them," in J. Hughes, J. Close, and A. La Greca (eds.), *Handbook of Psychological Services for Children and Adolescents,* New York: Oxford University Press.

Cavanaugh, D. A., J. Lippit, and O. Moyo (2000). "Resource Guide to Federal Policies Affecting Children's Social and Emotion Development and Their Readiness for School," in L. Huffman et al., *Off to a Good Start,* Report commissioned by the Child Mental Health Foundations and Agencies Network, New York.

Center for the Study of Social Policy (1996). *Systems Change at the Neighborhood Level: Creating Better Futures for Children, Youth, and Families,* Washington, DC, September.

Children's Cabinet (2002). *System of Care for Families with Very Young Children,* Birth to Five Committee Report Submitted to the Full Cabinet, Allegheny County, Pennsylvania, January.

Commonwealth of Pennsylvania, Department of Public Welfare (1997). *1915(b) Capitated Waiver Program Application: HealthChoices Program Expansion for Physical and Behavioral Health Services*, October.

Commonwealth of Pennsylvania, Department of Public Welfare (n.d.). Services Available, www.dpw. state.pa.us/general/program.asp.

Department of Health, Background Information (n.d.). http://www.health. state.pa.us/health/cwp.

Duggan, A., A. Windham, E. McFarlane, et al. (2000). "Hawaii's Healthy Start Program of Home Visiting for At-Risk Families: Evaluation of Family Identification, Family Engagement, and Service Delivery," *Pediatrics*, Vol. 105, No. 1, pp. 250–259.

Gortmaker, S. L., D. K. Walker, F. H. Jacobs, and H. Ruch-Ross (1982). "Parental Smoking and the Risk of Childhood Asthma," *American Journal of Public Health*, Vol. 76, No. 6, June.

Hanson, L., D. Deere, C. A. Lee, A. Lewin, and C. Seval (2001). *Key Principles in Providing Integrated Behavioral Health Services for Young Children and Their Families: The Starting Early Starting Smart Experience*, Washington, DC: Casey Family Programs and the U.S. Department of Health and Human Services, Substance Abuse and Mental Health Administration.

Health: Bureau of Health Statistics and Research (n.d.). http://www.health.state.pa.us/health/cwp/ view.asp?a=175&Q=228721.

Health Insurance Portability and Accountability Act of 1996 (1996). Pub. L. No. 104-191, 110 Stat. 1936 (codified as amended in scattered sections of 42 U.S.C.).

Healthy People 2010 (n.d.). http://www.healthypeople.gov/Document/HTML/Volume2/16MICH. html.

Healthy Start, Inc., http://trfn.clpgh.org/hspgh/chemically%20dep%20 mothers.html.

Hughes, R. G., T. L. Davis, and R. C. Reynolds (1995). "Assuring Children's Health as the Basis for Health Care Reform," *Health Affairs*, Vol. 14, No. 2.

Lewitt, E. M., L. S. Baker, H. Corman, and P. H. Shiono (1995). "The Direct Cost of Low Birthweight," *The Future of Children*, Vol. 5, No. 1, Los Altos, CA: The David and Lucille Packard Foundation.

Myoung, K., J. Ohls, and R. Cohen (2001). *Hunger in America 2001 Local Report Prepared from Greater Pittsburgh Food Bank—Allegheny County (8395), Final Report*, Princeton, NJ: Mathematica Policy Research, Inc., October.

The National Healthy Start Association: The Healthy Start Program (n.d.). http://www. healthystartassoc.org/hswpp6.html.

National Research Council and the Institute of Medicine (2000). J. P. Shonkoff and D. A. Phillips (eds.), *From Neurons to Neighborhoods: The Science of Early Childhood Development*, Committee on Integrating the Science of Early Childhood Development, Board on Children, Youth, and Families, Commission on Behavioral and Social Sciences and Education, Washington, DC: National Academy Press.

Nicholson, W. K., K. D. Frick, and N. R. Powe (2000). "Economic Burden of Hospitalizations for Preterm Labor in the United States," *Obstetrics and Gynecology*, Vol. 96, No. 1, July.

Pennsylvania Children's Health Insurance Program (2001). *Framework for Annual Report of State Children's Health Insurance Plans Under Title XXI of the Social Security Act*.

Pennsylvania Department of Health (July 10, 2001). *State Health Improvement Plan 2001–2005*.

Pennsylvania Department of Health (2003). http://www.health.state.pa.us/ stats, September.

Pennsylvania Office of Social Programs, *Medical Assistance Transportation Program* (n.d.). http://www.dpw.state.pa.us/osp/ospmatp.asp.

Powell, D., D. Fixsen, and G. Dunlap (2003). *Pathways to Service Utilization: A Synthesis of Evidence Relevant to Young Children with Challenging Behavior*, Tampa, FL: University of South Florida, Center for Evidence-Based Practice: Young Children with Challenging Behaviors, May 20.

Rogowski, J. (1998). "Cost Effectiveness of Care for Very Low Birth Weight Infants," *Pediatrics*, Vol. 102, No. 1, July.

Schorr, L. B. (1997). *Common Purpose: Strengthening Families and Neighborhoods to Rebuild America*, New York: Anchor Books, Doubleday.

Sunyer, J., M. Saez, C. Murillo, J. Castellsague, F. Martinez, and J. M. Anto (1993). "Air Pollution and Emergency Room Admissions for Chronic Obstructive Pulmonary Disease: A Five-Year Study," *American Journal of Epidemiology,* Vol. 137, No. 7, April.

Tobacco Free Allegheny (n.d.). http://www.tobaccofreeallegheny.com// healthcare.html (accessed February 10, 2004).

U.S. Department of Health and Human Services (n.d.). http://odphp.osophs.dhhs.gov/pubs/ healthycommunities (accessed July 26, 2004).